Spanish for Nurses

Rudy Valenzuela

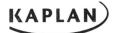

KAPLAN

PUBLISHING

New York

© 2009 Rudy Valenzuela.

Published by Kaplan Publishing, a division of Kaplan, Inc.
1 Liberty Plaza, 24th Floor
New York, NY 10006

Printed in the United States of America

10   9   8   7   6   5   4   3   2   1

ISBN-13: 978-1-4277-9976-0

Kaplan Publishing books are available at special quantity discounts to use for sales promotions, employee premiums, or educational purposes. Please email our Special Sales Department to order or for more information at kaplan publishing@kaplan.com, or write to Kaplan Publishing, 1 Liberty Plaza, 24th Floor, New York, NY 10006.

Contents

Dedication

A mi padre.

About the Author

Br. Valenzuela is the President/CEO of FSP Health
Ministries, a non-profit organization that sponsors
Camillus Health Center in San Luis, AZ., and Clínica
Santa Maria de Guadalupe in San Luis, Rio Colorado,
Sonora Mexico. He is a family nurse practitioner and a
Friar of the Sick Poor, a congregation of religious men
in the Catholic Church.

Acknowledgment

Special thanks to Melisa Mora for her assistance
during this project.

Introduction

To talk about language is to talk about culture. Culture influences every aspect of our lives, even the way we communicate. Therefore communicating in one's own language of preference is important. In the United States, Spanish-speaking residents are the fastest-growing segment of the population. For healthcare professionals in the United States today, the ability to communicate in the language of our patients is essential to the care we give.

➤ TARGET AUDIENCE

This book was written for healthcare professionals, particularly nurses, to promote communication with an ever-expanding, ethnically and linguistically diverse population. Created for nurses, by a nurse, it is intended to assist with the collection of basic healthcare information from Spanish-speaking patients and clients. The book is designed primarily for use in settings where the need for on-the-spot communication is greatest: emergency departments, urgent care centers, and maternity wards, as well as in ambulatory and outpatient settings, including (but not limited to) physicians' offices, diagnostic centers, and outpatient surgery centers.

➤ HOW TO USE THIS BOOK

The book contains an introduction to Spanish essentials, eight additional chapters based on the medical care settings just mentioned, and a glossary. Each chapter presents the most commonly asked questions for that specific setting. All questions are designed to permit the practicioner to extrapolate basic answers in a direct- or closed-question format. For example, the nurse may want to know whether the patient or client has pain. We present a simple way of asking the question so that the client may respond in the affirmative or the negative: *¿Tiene dolor?* (tee-'eh-neh doh-'lohr) (Do you have pain?)

To this question, the patient has only the options of responding with *si (see) (yes)* or with *no (noh) (no)*. To further investigate the location of the pain, the nurse may ask, *¿Le duele el estómago?* (leh 'dweh-leh ehl ehs-'toh-mah-goh) (Does your stomach hurt?). This format encourages the use of specific information. It also elicits facts, calls for one- to two-word answers, and is more easily understandable by non-Spanish speaking healthcare professionals. This book is not a substitute for the valuable services of a professional interpreter, and when in doubt, the practicioner should request such assistance. The book is designed to enable basic communication between healthcare provider and patient in crisis situations when an interpreter is not available.

Pronunciation Guide

It is suggested that you go through this pronunciation guide before tackling the rest of the book, to make it easier for you to pronounce the different phrases presented in the rest of the book.

Spanish is easy to pronounce because it is remarkably consistent, compared with English.

The five vowels have the following sounds:

A   as in *father, alms, ah*

E   as in *better, leg, send*

I   as *e* sound in *he, peel, dream*

O   as in *most, coast, float*

U   as in *soup, flute, food*

Only the *u* is a bit tricky at times: if it follows a *q*, you do not pronounce it at all, and the same is true if it is between a *g* and an *e*, or between a *g* and an *i*, unless there are two little dots over the *u* (*ü*) to tell you that in that particular word you should pronounce it.

Consonants have pretty much the same sounds as they have in English, with a few exceptions:

C   sounds like *c* in *cat* before *a, o,* or *u,* and before most consonants. Before *e* or *i* it sounds like *s* in *sun*.
When two *c*s appear together in a word, the first sounds like *c* in *cat* and the second sounds like *s* (*acción*). When *c* is followed by an *h*, the two letters together are pronounced like the *ch* in English (as in *chicken*).

G	sounds like *g* in *goat* before *a, o,* or *u,* but before *e* or *i* it sounds like *h* as in *hat*
J	sounds like *h* in *ha*
H	silent
LL	sounds like *y* in *yawn*
Ñ	sounds like *ny* in *canyon*
QU	sounds like *k* in *key*
R	sounds like *r* in *car;* as first letter in word, pronounced rolled like RR
RR	rolled *r*

➤ *SYLLABLE STRESS*

In the pronunciation keys underneath each word and phrase, there will be marks (′) that look like apostrophes. These are stress marks, placed in front of the syllables that should be emphasized. In most words, the emphasis goes on the next to last syllable. Words with that pattern are written without an accent mark. When you see an accent, put the emphasis there. Of course all these rules have to have exceptions. Spanish words that end with a consonant (such as with the letter *r*) usually have the accent on the last syllable. There's even an exception to that. Words that end in *s* and words ending in vowels have the emphasis on the next-to-last syllable, unless an accent mark tells you otherwise. Thus *dolor* (pain), *calor* (heat), and *Doctor* (Doctor) should be spoken with the emphasis at the end of the word.

Spanish Essentials

1

➤ GREETINGS

Spanish-speaking people have both a formal and an informal way of addressing each other. *Usted* (*oo-'stehd*) and *tú* (*too*) both mean *you*, but their uses differ in the following way: *Usted* (*oo-'stehd*) is used for a person who is older or who has a higher level of authority or education, such as a healthcare professional. The more informal *tú* (*too*) is used among peers and friends, and with younger people. Given that the Hispanic population is mostly younger than the rest of the U.S. population, the informal *tú* (*too*) is more often encountered. An example of the use of formal address would be *¿Cómo está usted hoy?* (*'koh-moh eh-'stah oo-'stehd 'oh-yee*) (*How are you today?*). When in doubt, always ask the patient how he or she prefers to be addressed: *¿Prefiere que le llame de usted?* (*preh-fee-'eh-reh keh leh 'yah-meh deh oo-'stehd*) (*Would you prefer that I address you as* **usted**?)

Another respectful form of address among Spanish-speaking people is the use of *Don* (*dohn*) (literally, *mister*), or *Doña* (*doh-'nyah*) (literally, *madam*), followed by the person's first name, as in the following example: *Buenos días, Doña María* (*'bwehn-ohs 'dee-ahs 'doh-nyah mah-'ree-ah*) (*Good morning, Madam Maria*).

The purposes of attempting to communicate in somebody else's language are manifold: obtaining information, appreciating the cultural values of the other person, and gaining trust, among others. Most Hispanic people appreciate it when the healthcare provider starts the conversation about something other than the person involved in the interview. It is therefore important that the healthcare professional follow the initial greeting (such as *good morning*) with small talk, such as asking about the patient's family: *¿Cómo está la familia?* (*'koh-moh eh-'stah lah fah-'mee-lee-ah) (How is your family?)* The usual answer will be *está bien, gracias (eh-'stah bee-'ehn 'grah-see-ahs) (They are doing fine, thank you)*. If the patient or client inquiries about your family (a usual sign of etiquette), you can respond with the same answer: *Está bien, gracias (eh-'stah bee-'ehn 'grah-see-ahs)*.

Following are some examples of greetings most commonly used by Spanish-speaking people. The examples follow the usual outline for greeting another person and for introducing oneself to that person.

Good morning.
Buenos días.
(boo-'eh-nohs 'dee-ahs)

Good afternoon.
Buenas tardes.
(boo-'eh-nahs 'tahr-dehs)

Good evening./Good night. (usually said as a greeting after the sun sets, and also used as a good-bye at night)
Buenas noches.
(boo-'eh-nahs 'noh-chehs)

Hello.
Hola.
('oh-lah)

My name is (name).
Me llamo _____.
(meh 'yah-moh)

I am (name).
Yo soy _____.
(yoh 'so-ee)

How are you? (formal)
¿Cómo está usted?
('koh-moh ehs-'tah oo-'stehd)

How are you? (informal)
¿Cómo estás tú?
('koh-moh ehs-'tahs too)

How are you? (another form of the informal)
¿Cómo estás?
('koh-moh ehs-'tahs)

Have a good morning/day.
Que pase buenos días.
(keh 'pah-seh boo-'eh-nohs 'dee-ahs)

Have a good evening.
Que pase buenas tardes.
(keh 'pah-seh boo-'eh-nahs tahr-'dehs)

Have a good night.
Que pase buenas noches.
(keh 'pah-seh boo-'eh-nahs 'noh-chehs)

Good-bye.
Adiós.
(ah-dee-'ohs)

See you later.
Hasta luego.
(ah-'stah loo-'eh-goh)

INDEFINITE ARTICLES IN SPANISH

It is important to remember the different use of indirect articles in Spanish (a, an). They show number and gender, as in *una herida* (a wound), *unas mujeres* (some women), *un hogar* (a home), *unos hombres* (some men).

DEFINITE ARTICLES IN SPANISH

Definite articles (the) also show number and gender, as in *la herida* (the wound), *las mujeres* (the women), *el lugar* (the place), and *los hombres* (the men). Spanish, however, sometimes does not use definite articles where English does, as in the following material.

I am a (male) nurse.
Soy enfermero.
(so-ee ehn-fehr-'meh-roh)

I am a (female) nurse.
Soy enfermera.
(so-ee ehn-fehr-'meh-rah)

I am a physician.
Soy médico.
(so-ee 'meh-dee-koh)

I am a paramedic.
Soy paramédico.
(so-ee pah-rah-'meh-dee-koh)

I am an assistant.
Soy asistente.
(so-ee ah-'sees-tehn-teh)

I am a technician.
Soy técnico.
(so-ee 'tehk-nee-koh)

I am a secretary.
Soy secretaria.
(so-ee seh-'kreh-tah-ree-ah)

COMMON RESPONSES

Yes.
Sí.
(see)

No.
No.
(noh)

Please.
Por favor.
(pohr fah-'bohr)

Thank you.
Gracias
('grah-see-ahs)

Excuse me.
Con permiso.
(kohn pehr-'mee-soh)

I don't understand.
No entiendo.
(noh ehn-'tee-ehn-doh)

➤ *NUMBERS*

Following is a list of numbers from 0 to 100. Remember that most numbers in Spanish do not change, except for **uno** *('oo-noh)* *(one)*. The number one changes form when preceded by a masculine singular noun, e.g., **un gato** *(one cat)*. The word for one hundred is **cien** *(see-'ehn)*, but **ciento** *(see-'ehn-toh)* is used to combine with another number, as in **ciento uno** *(see-'ehn-toh 'oo-noh)* *(one hundred one)*.

0
Cero
('seh-roh)

1
Uno
('oo-noh)

2
Dos
(dohs)

3
Tres
(trehs)

4
Cuatro
('kwah-troh)

5
Cinco
('seehn-koh)

6
Seis
('seh-ees)

7
Siete
(see'eh-teh)

8
Ocho
('oh-choh)

9
Nueve
(noo-'eh-beh)

10
Diez
('dee-ehs)

11
Once
('ohn-seh)

12
Doce
('doh-seh)

13
Trece
('treh-seh)

1

14
Catorce
(kah-'tohr-seh)

15
Quince
('keen-seh)

16
Dieciséis
(dee-ehs-ee-'seh-ees)

17
Diecisiete
(dee-ehs-ee-see-'eh-teh)

18
Dieciocho
(dee-ehs-ee-'oh-choh)

19
Diecinueve
(dee-ehs-ee-noo-'eh-beh)

20
Veinte
(beh-'een-teh)

30
Treinta
(treh-'een-tah)

40
Cuarenta
(kwah-'rehn-tah)

50
Cincuenta
(seen-'kwehn-tah)

60
Sesenta
(seh-'sehn-tah)

70
Setenta
(seh-'tehn-tah)

80
Ochenta
(oh-'chehn-tah)

90
Noventa
(noh-'behn-tah)

100
Cien
(see-'ehn)

200
Doscientos
(dohs-see-'ehn-tohs)

300
Trescientos
(treh-see-'ehn-tohs)

400
Cuatrocientos
('kwah-troh-see-'ehn-tohs)

1

500
Quinientos
(keen-ee-'ehn-tohs)

600
Seiscientos
(seh-ees-see-'ehn-tohs)

700
Setecientos
(see-eh-teh-see-'ehn-tohs)

800
Ochocientos
(oh-choh-see-'ehn-tohs)

900
Novecientos
(noh-beh-see-'ehn-tohs)

1000
Mil
(meel)

2000
Dos mil
(dohs-meel)

3000
Tres mil
(trehs-meel)

and so forth

1,000,000
Un millón
(oon mee-'yohn)

You form numbers by adding the names of the component numbers together with **y**. For example, 31: **treinta y uno** *(treh-'een-tah ee 'oo-noh)* *(thirty and one)*; 28: **ventiocho** *(beh-'een-teh ee 'oh-choh)*; 192: **ciento noventa y dos** *(see-'ehn toh noh-'behn-tah ee dohs)*; 1159: **mil ciento cincuenta y nueve** *(mel see-'ehn toh seen-'kwehn-tah ee noo-'eh-beh)*.

First
Primero
(pree-'meh-roh)

Second
Segundo
(seh-'goon-doh)

Third
Tercero
(tehr-'seh-roh)

Fourth
Cuarto
('kwahr-toh)

Fifth
Quinto
('keen-toh)

Sixth
Sexto
('sehks-toh)

Seventh
Séptimo
(s'ehp-tee-moh)

1

Eighth
Octavo
(ohk-'tah-boh)

Ninth
Noveno
(noh-'beh-noh)

Tenth
Décimo
('deh-see-moh)

➤ *FAMILY MEMBERS*

One's relationships with others are important among Spanish-speaking people, so it is important to become acquainted with the Spanish terms for family relations. Most of the time patients will want to refer to a family health history, or they may rely on a relative for health or demographic data. For example, an older female adult may rely on the daughter-in-law for assistance with activities of daily living, medication administration, or transportation. Following is a list of the most commonly used family terms:

Father/Daddy
Padre/Papá
('pah-dreh/pah-'pah)

Mother/Mama
Madre/Mamá
('mah-dreh/mah-'mah)

Brother
Hermano
(ehr-'mah-noh)

Sister
Hermana
(ehr-'mah-nah)

Grandfather
Abuelo
(ah-'bweh-loh)

Grandmother
Abuela
(ah-'bweh-lah)

Grandson
Nieto
(nee-'eh-toh)

Granddaughter
Nieta
(nee-'eh-tah)

Uncle
Tío
('tee-oh)

Aunt
Tía
('tee-ah)

Cousin
Primo/Prima
('pree-moh/'pree-mah)

Niece
Sobrina
(soh-'bree-nah)

1

Nephew
Sobrino
(soh-'bree-noh)

Father-in-law
Suegro
('sweh-groh)

Mother-in-law
Suegra
('sweh-grah)

Brother-in-law
Cuñado
(koo-'nyah-doh)

Sister-in-law
Cuñada
(koo-'nyah-dah)

Stepfather
Padrastro
(pah-'drahs-troh)

Stepmother
Madrastra
(mah-'drahs-trah)

Stepson
Hijastro
(ee-'hahs-troh)

Stepdaughter
Hijastra
(ee-'hahs-trah)

Great-grandfather
Bisabuelo
(bees-ah-'bweh-loh)

Great-grandmother
Bisabuela
(bees-ah-'bweh-lah)

Great-grandson
Bisnieto
(bees-nee-'eh-toh)

Great-granddaughter
Bisnieta
(bees-nee-'eh-tah)

The relationship of godparents and godchildren is important to most Spanish-speaking people. This relationship is acquired when the parents of the child ask friends to become the child's godparents at a religious ceremony such as a baptism. Following are some of the names that distinguish this particular relationship. It is important to recognize these names, as godparents and godchildren may at times be considered next of kin, especially on occasions when a child is hospitalized, and the godparents wish to visit the sick child.

Godfather
Padrino
(pah-'dree-noh)

Godmother
Madrina
(mah-'dree-nah)

Goddaughter
Ahijada
(ah-ee-'hah-dah)

1

Godson
Ahijado
(ah-ee-'hah-doh)

Compadre
Compadre
(kohm-'pah-dreh)

➤ DATE AND TIME

Following are some examples of the most commonly used date and time questions and answers.

TIME

What time is it?
¿Qué horas son?/¿Qué hora es?
(keh 'oh-rahs sohn/keh 'oh-rah ehs)

It is six o'clock.
Son las seis.
(sohn lahs 'seh-ees)

It is seven forty five in the morning
Son las siete y cuarenta y cinco.
(sohn lahs see-'eh-teh ee kwah-'rehn-tah ee 'seehn-koh)

It is midnight.
Es medianoche.
(ehs meh-dee-ah-'noh-cheh)

It is noon.
Es mediodía.
(ehs meh-dee-oh-'dee-ah)

It is ten fifty five.
Son las diez y cincuenta y cinco.
(sohn las dee-'ehs ee seen-'kwehn-tah ee 'seehn-koh)

What day is it?
¿Qué día es?
(keh 'dee-ah ehs)

What month is it?
¿Qué mes es?
(keh mehs ehs)

What year is it?
¿Qué año es?
(keh 'ah-nyoh ehs)

DAYS OF THE WEEK

Monday
Lunes
('loo-nehs)

Tuesday
Martes
('mahr-tehs)

Wednesday
Miércoles
(mee-'ehr-koh-lehs)

Thursday
Jueves
('hweh-behs)

1

Friday
Viernes
(bee-'ehr-nehs)

Saturday
Sábado
('sah-bah-doh)

Sunday
Domingo
(doh-'meen-goh)

Today is Friday.
Hoy es viernes.
(ohy ehs bee-'ehr-nehs)

Tomorrow will be Monday.
Mañana es lunes.
(mah-'nyah-nah ehs 'loo-nehs)

Yesterday was Thursday.
Ayer fue jueves.
(ah-'yehr fweh 'hweh-behs)

DAYS OF THE MONTH

The most common way of naming the days of the month (and the easiest to remember) is to use the ordinal number, as previously reviewed. For example:

First
Primero
(pree-'meh-roh)

Second
Segundo
(seh-'goon-doh)

Third
Tercero
(tehr-'seh-roh)

Fourth
Cuarto
('kwahr-toh)

Fifth
Quinto
('keen-toh)

Sixth
Sexto
('sehks-toh)

Seventh
Séptimo
('sehp-tee-moh)

Eighth
Octavo
(ohk-'tah-boh)

Ninth
Noveno
(noh-'beh-noh)

Tenth
Décimo
('deh-see-moh)

Eleventh
Undécimo
(oon-'deh-see-moh)

Twelfth
Duodécimo
(doo-oh-'deh-see-moh)

Thirteenth
Decimotercero
(deh-see-moh-tehr-'seh-roh)

Fourteenth
Decimocuarto
(deh-see-moh-'kwahr-toh)

Fifteenth
Decimoquinto
(deh-see-moh-'keen-toh)

Sixteenth
Decimosexto
(deh-see-moh-'sehks-toh)

Seventeenth
Decimoséptimo
(deh-see-moh-'sehp-tee-moh)

Eighteenth
Decimoctavo
(deh-see-mohk-'tah-boh)

Nineteenth
Decimonoveno
(deh-see-moh-noh-'beh-noh)

Twentieth
Vigésimo
(bee-'heh-see-moh)

Thirtieth
Trigésimo
(tree-'heh-see-moh)

MONTHS OF THE YEAR

January
Enero
(eh-'neh-roh)

February
Febrero
(feh-'brehr-oh)

March
Marzo
('mahr-soh)

April
Abril
(ah-'breel)

1

May
Mayo
('mah-yoh)

June
Junio
('hoo-nee-oh)

July
Julio
('hoo-lee-oh)

August
Agosto
(ah-'goh-stoh)

September
Septiembre
(sehp-tee-'ehm-breh)

October
Octubre
(ohk-'too-breh)

November
Noviembre
(noh-vee-'ehm-breh)

December
Diciembre
(dee-see-'ehm-breh)

Today is the first of November.
Hoy es el primero de noviembre.
('oh-ee ehs ehl pree-'meh-roh deh noh-vee-'ehm-breh)

Yesterday was the 23rd of June.
Ayer fué el veintitrés de junio.
(ah-'yehr fweh ehl beh-een-tee-'trehs deh 'hoo-nee-oh)

YEARS

In dates, **ciento** (*'see- 'ehn' toh*) is used to designate the century; e.g., 1283: **mil doscientos ochenta y tres** (*meel dohs-see-'ehn-tohs oh-'chehn-tah ee trehs*) (literally "one thousand two hundred and eighty-three").

Most Spanish-speaking countries determine a date by first naming the day, then the day of the month, the month, and finally the year, e.g. **Lunes, doce de agosto de mil novecientos noventa y siete** (*'loo-nehs, 'doh-seh deh ah-'goh-stoh deh meel noh-beh-see-'ehn-tohs noh-'behn-tah ee see'eh-teh*) (Monday, the twelfth of August, 1997).

When were you born?
¿Cuándo nació?
('kwahn-doh nah-see-'oh)

I was born on May 2, 1942.
Nací el dos de mayo de mil novecientos cuarenta y dos. (nah-'see ehl dohs deh 'mah-yoh deh meel noh-beh-see-'ehn-tohs kwah-'rehn-tah ee dohs)

When were you married?
¿Cuándo se casó?
('kwahn-doh seh kah-'soh)

I married on December 4, 1965.
Me casé el cuatro de diciembre de mil novecientos sesenta y cinco. (meh kah-'seh ehl 'kwah-troh deh dee-see-'ehm-breh deh meel noh-beh-see-'ehn-tohs seh-'sehn-tah ee 'seehn-koh)

At the Clinic

2

This chapter presents situations that arise during the usual first encounter between the healthcare provider and the Spanish-speaking client. While particularly useful in the walk-in clinic, it applies to a variety of healthcare settings. This dialogue presents the most commonly used questions and answers. It presents various ways of asking the same question so that the healthcare professional can communicate with monolingual Spanish speakers in a variety of ways.

Most Hispanic people, as in many other cultures, are highly respectful of healthcare personnel. One must be careful to treat Hispanic patients with the same respect. A respectful, friendly gesture will go a long way when serving the Hispanic population. You may try this exercise when you first start using this book. Choose a greeting of your choice, for example, *Buenos días ('bwehn-ohs 'dee-ahs)*, and then add another question related to the client's family, e.g. *¿Cómo está su esposa (esposo)? (ehs-'poh-sah / ehs-'poh-soh)* (how is your wife [husband]?) You will be able to see the immediate response of the client, and you will build trust as you continue with the task of caring for others. As you build your confidence in speaking Spanish, try adding other questions related to the client's interest, for example, *¿Donde nació usted? ('dohn-deh*

2

nah-see-'oh oo-'stehd) (Where were you born?) or *¿Cuántos nietos tiene?* (*'kwahn-tohs nee-'eh-tohs tee-'eh-neh*) (How many grandchildren do you have?). These questions, taken for granted in regular conversation, can open the door to more holistic, culturally competent care.

➤ *FRONT OFFICE*

Remember the greetings and other basic terms you learned in the previous chapter. Conversations usually start with a simple greeting, such as *Buenos días* (*'bwehn-ohs 'dee-ahs*) (Good morning).

Reason for Visit

How can I help you?
¿En que puedo ayudarle?
(ehn keh poo-'eh-doh ah-yoo-'dahr-leh)

Good Morning. Tell me the reason for your visit.
Buenos días. Dígame la razón de su visita.
('bweh-nohs 'dee-ahs. dee-gah-meh lah rah-'sohn deh soo bee-'see-tah)

What brings you to the office today?
¿A qué viene a la oficina hoy?
(ah keh bee-'eh-neh ah lah oh-fee-'see-nah 'oh-ee)

Possible Answers:

I'm here to see the doctor.
Vengo a ver al doctor.
('behn-goh ah behr ahl dohk-'tohr)

I'm here to have my blood drawn.
Vengo a sacarme sangre.
('behn-goh ah sah-'kahr-meh 'sahn-greh)

I'm here for my annual physical.
Vengo a mi examen anual.
('behn-goh ah mee ehk-'sah-mehn ah-nuh-'ahl)

I need to see the nurse.
Necesito ver a la enfermera.
(neh-seh-'see-toh behr ah lah ehn-fehr-'meh-rah)

I need a prescription.
Necesito una receta (prescripción).
(neh-seh-'see-toh 'oo-nah reh-'seh-tah (preh-skreep-see-'ohn))

I'm here to pick up my prescription.
Vengo por mi receta (prescripción).
('behn-goh pohr mee reh-'seh-tah (preh-skreep-see-'ohn))

I'm here to get my referral.
Vengo por mi referimiento.
('behn-goh pohr mee reh-fehr-ee-mee-'ehn-toh)

I'm here to drop off some papers.
Vengo a entregar unos papeles.
('behn-goh ah ehn-treh-'gahr 'oo-nohs pah-'pehl-ehs)

Insurance

Do you have insurance?
¿Tiene aseguranza (seguro médico)?
(tee-'eh-neh ah-seh-goo-'rahn-sah (seh-'goo-roh 'meh-dee-koh))

2

What kind of insurance do you have?

¿Qué tipo de aseguranza tiene?

(keh' tee-poh de hah-seh-goor-'ahn-sah tee-'eh-neh)

Do you have your insurance card?

¿Tiene su tarjeta de aseguranza?

(tee-'eh-neh soo tahr-'heh-tah deh ah-seh-goo-'rahn-sah)

How long have you had it?

¿Desde cuándo la tiene?

('dehs-deh 'kwahn-doh lah tee-'eh-neh)

When did it expire?

¿Cuándo se le venció?

('kwahn-doh seh leh behn-see-'oh)

Do you have any other kind of insurance?

¿Tiene algún otro tipo de aseguranza?

(tee-'eh-neh ahl-'goohn 'oh-troh 'tee-poh deh ah-seh-goo-'rahn-sah)

What is your co-pay?

¿Cuál es su co-pago?

('kwal ehs soo koh-'pah-goh)

What is your social security number?

¿Cuál es su número de seguro social?

('kwahl ehs soo 'noo-meh-roh deh seh-'goo-roh soh-see-'ahl)

Do you have your driver's license?

¿Tiene su licencia de manejar?

(tee-'eh-neh soo lee-'sehn-see-ah deh mah-neh-'hahr)

I have Medicare.

Tengo Medicare.

('tehn-goh 'meh-dee-kehr)

I do not have insurance.
No tengo aseguranza.
(noh 'tehn-goh ah-seh-goo-'rahn-sah)

I have private insurance.
Tengo aseguranza privada.
('tehn-goh ah-seh-goo-'rahn-sah pree-'bah-dah)

My co-pay is twenty dollars.
Mi co-pago es veinte dólares.
(meek koh-'pah-goh ehs beh-'een-teh 'doh-lah-rehs)

My social security number is _____.
Mi número de seguro social es _____.
(mee 'noo-meh-roh deh seh-'goo-roh soh-see-'ahl ehs)

I lost my insurance card.
Perdí mi tarjeta de aseguranza.
(pehr-'dee mee tahr-'heh-tah deh ah-seh-goo-'rahn-sah)

Healthcare Provider

Who is your doctor?
¿Quién es su doctor?
(kee-'ehn ehs soo dohk-'tohr)

Who is your specialist?
¿Quién es su especialista?
(kee-'ehn ehs soo ehs-peh-see-ah-'lees-tah)

I'm here to see Dr. _____.
Vengo a ver al Doctor _____.
('behn-goh ah behr ahl dohk-'tohr)

Cardiologist
Cardiólogo
(kahr-dee-'oh-loh-goh)

Orthopedist
Ortopedista
(ohr-toh-peh-'dees-tah)

Pulmonologist
Pulmonólogo
(pool-moh-'noh-loh-goh)

Podiatrist
Podiatra
(poh-dee-'ah-trah)

Internist
Internista
(een-tehr-'nees-tah

Surgeon
Cirujano
(see-roo-'hah-noh)

Nephrologist
Nefrólogo
(neh-'froh-loh-goh)

Nurse
Enfermera(o)
(ehn-fehr-'meh-rah / ehn-fehr-'meh-roh)

Advanced practice nurse
Enfermera(o) de práctica avanzada
(ehn-fehr-'meh-rah / roh deh 'prahk-tee-kah ah-vahn-'sah-dah)

➤ *TRIAGE*

Personal Information

Tell me your name, please.
Dígame su nombre, por favor.
('dee-gah-meh soo 'nohm-breh, pohr fah-'bohr)

Slower, please.
Más despacio, por favor.
(mahs dehs-'pah-see-oh, pohr fah-'bohr)

What is your date of birth?
¿Cuál es su fecha de nacimiento?
('kwahl ehs soo 'feh-chah deh nah-see-mee-'ehn-toh)

When where you born?
¿Cuándo nació?
('kwahn-doh nah-see-'oh)

How old are you?
¿Cuántos años tiene?
('kwahn-tohs 'ah-nyohs tee-'eh-neh)

How old are you?
¿Qué edad tiene?
(keh eh-'dad tee-'eh-neh)

I am sixty years old.
Tengo sesenta años.
('tehn-goh seh-'sehn-tah 'ah-nyohs)

He is two months old.
Él tiene dos meses.
(ehl tee-'eh-neh dohs 'meh-sehs)

She is going to be thirty next month.

Ella va a cumplir treinta años el próximo mes.

('eh-yah bah ah koom-'pleer treh-'een-tah 'ah-nyohs ehl 'prohk-see-moh mehs)

Where do you live?

¿Dónde vive?

('dohn-deh 'bee-beh)

I live in Long Beach.

Vivo en Long Beach.

('bee-boh ehn long beach)

I live in an apartment.

Vivo en un apartamento.

('bee-boh ehn oon ah-pahr-tah-'mehn-toh)

I live with my mother.

Vivo con mi madre (mamá).

('bee-boh kohn mee 'mah-dreh)(mah-'mah)

I live with my son.

Vivo con mi hijo.

('bee-boh kohn mee 'ee-hoh)

What is your address?

¿Cuál es su dirección?

(kwahl ehs soo dee-rehk-see-'ohn)

How long have you lived there?

¿Cuánto tiempo ha vivido allí?

('kwahn-toh tee-'ehm-poh ah bee-'bee-doh ah-'yee)

What is your phone number?

¿Cuál es su número de teléfono?

('kwahl ehs soo 'noo-meh-roh deh teh-'leh-foh-noh)

My phone number is _____.
Mi número de teléfono es _____.
(mee 'noo-meh-roh deh teh-'leh-foh-noh ehs)

What do you work as?
¿En qué trabaja?
(ehn keh trah-'bah-hah)

What do you do?
¿A qué se dedica?
(ah keh seh deh-'dee-kah)

I am a carpenter.
Soy carpintero.
(soy kahr-peen-'teh-roh)

Plumber
Plomero
(ploh-'meh-roh)

Electrician
Electricista
(eh-lehk-tree-'sees-tah)

Clerk
Cajera
(kah-'heh-rah)

Therapist
Terapista
(teh-rah-'pees-tah)

I work in the fields.
Trabajo en el campo.
(trah-'bah-hoh ehn ehl 'kahm-poh)

I work in construction.
Trabajo en construcción.
(trah-'bah-hoh ehn kohn-strook-see-'ohn)

I am an assistant.
Soy asistente.
(soy ah-'sees-tehn-teh)

I am a cook.
Soy cocinera.
(soy koh-see-'neh-rah)

I am a physician.
Soy un médico.
(soy oon 'meh-dee-koh)

I clean houses.
Limpio casas.
('leem-pee-oh 'kah-sahs)

I drive a taxi.
Manejo un taxi.
(mah-'neh-hoh oon 'tahk-see)

I am a student.
Soy estudiante.
(soy ehs-too-dee-'ahn-teh)

Are you married?
¿Es casado(a)?
(ehs kah-'sah-doh / kah-'sah-dah)

Widow (widower)?
¿Viuda(o)?
(vee-oo-dah / vee-oo-doh)

Divorced?
¿Divorciado(a)?
(dee-bohr-see-'ah-doh /dee-bohr-see-'ah-dah)

Separated?
¿Separado(a)?
(seh-pah-'rah-doh /seh-pah-'rah-dah)

Chief Complaint(s)

Questions are the same as in the Front Office section (page 26).

Most common chief complaints/answers:

I have chest pain.
Tengo dolor de pecho.
('tehn-goh doh-'lohr deh 'peh-choh)

I have a headache.
Tengo dolor de cabeza.
('tehn-goh doh-'lohr deh kah-'beh-sah)

I have a stomachache.
Me duele el estómago.
(meh doo-'eh-leh ehl ehs-'toh-mah-goh)

I can't breathe.
No puedo respirar.
(noh poo-'eh-doh rehs-pee-'rahr)

I am itching.
Tengo comezón.
('tehn-goh koh-meh-'sohn)

2

I have fever.
Tengo fiebre (calentura).
('tehn-goh fee-'eh-breh (cah-lehn-'too-rah))

I feel weak.
Me siento débil.
(meh see-'ehn-toh 'deh-beel)

I have a toothache.
Me duele un diente.
(meh doo-'eh-leh oon dee-'ehn-teh)

Pediatrics

He / she has an earache.
Le duele un oído.
(leh doo-'eh-leh oon oh-'ee-doh)

He / she has a sore throat.
Le duele la garganta.
(leh doo-'eh-leh lah gahr-'gahn-tah)

He / she won't stop crying.
No para de llorar.
(noh 'pah-rah deh yoh-'rahr)

He / she has a fever.
Tiene fiebre.
(tee-'eh-neh fee-'eh-breh)

Vital Signs

How much do you weigh?
¿Cuánto pesa?
('kwahn-toh 'peh-sah)

Allow me to take your temperature.
Permítame tomarle la temperatura.
(pehr-'mee-tah-meh toh-'mahr-leh lah tehm-peh-rah-'too-rah)

Open your mouth.
Abra la boca.
('ah-brah lah 'boh-kah)

Close your mouth.
Cierre la boca.
(see-'eh-reh lah 'boh-kah)

In your ear.
En su oído.
(ehn soo oh-'ee-doh)

Allow me to take your pulse.
Permítame tomarle el pulso.
(pehr-'mee-tah-meh toh-'mahr-leh ehl 'pool-soh)

Allow me to take your breathing.
Permítame tomarle la respiración.
(pehr-'mee-tah-meh toh-'mahr-leh lah rehs-pee-rah-see-'ohn)

Allow me to take your blood pressure.
Permítame tomarle la presión sanguínea.
(pehr-'mee-tah-meh toh-'mahr-leh lah preh-'see-ohn sahn-'gee-neh-ah)

2

Do you have pain?

¿Tiene dolor?

(tee-'eh-neh doh-'lohr)

If zero means no pain, and ten means the greatest pain you ever had,

Si cero es ningún dolor, y diez el dolor más fuerte que haya tenido

(see 'seh-roh ehs neen-'goon doh-'lohr, ee 'dee-ehs ehl doh-'lohr mahs 'fwehr-teh keh 'hah-yah teh-'nee-doh)

What number do you give your pain?

¿Qué numero le da a su dolor?

(keh 'noo-meh-roh leh dah ah soo doh-'lohr)

How much pain do you have?

¿Cuánto dolor tiene?

(kuh-'ahn-toh doh-'lohr tee-'eh-neh)

Little

Poco

('poh-koh)

Moderate

Moderado

(moh-deh-'rah-doh)

A lot.

Mucho

('moo-choh)

➤ PAST MEDICAL HISTORY

Do you have high blood pressure?

¿Tiene presión alta?

(tee-'eh-neh preh-see-'ohn 'ahl-tah)

Do you have diabetes?
¿Tiene diabetes?
(tee-'eh-neh dee-ah-'beh-tehs)

Cancer?
¿Cáncer?
('kahn-sehr)

Heart disease?
¿Enfermedades del corazón?
(ehn-fehr-meh-'dah-dehs dehl koh-rah-'sohn)

Embolism?
¿Embolia?
(ehm-boh-'lee-ah)

Stroke?
¿Ataque súbito y agudo?
(ah-'tah-keh 'soo-bee-toh ee ah-'goo-doh)

Seizures / epilepsy?
¿Epilepsia?
(eh-pee-'lehp-see-ah)

Surgeries?
¿Cirugias?
(see-roo-'hee-ahs)

Medications

Do you take any pills / medicine?
¿Toma algún medicamento?
('toh-mah ahl-'goon meh-dee-kah-'mehn-toh)

Medicine?
¿Medicina?
(meh-dee-'see-nah)

What pills / medicine do you take?
¿Qué medicamentos toma?
(keh meh-dee-kah-'mehn-tohs 'toh-mah)

Do you take pills for high blood pressure?
¿Toma medicamento para la presión alta?
('toh-mah meh-dee-kah-'mehn-toh 'pah-rah lah preh-see-'ohn 'ahl-tah)

Do you take pills for diabetes?
¿Toma medicamento para la diabetes?
('toh-mah meh-dee-kah-'mehn-toh 'pah-rah lah dee-ah-'beh-tehs)

Do you take pills for your heart?
¿Toma medicamentos para el corazón?
('toh-mah meh-dee-kah-'mehn-tohs 'pah-rah ehl koh-rah-'sohn)

Do you take pills for your stomach?
¿Toma medicamento para el estómago?
('toh-mah meh-dee-kah-'mehn-toh 'pah-rah ehl eh-'stoh-mah-goh)

Do you take pills for anemia?
¿Toma medicamento para la anemia?
('toh-mah meh-dee-kah-'mehn-toh 'pah-rah lah ah-'neh-mee-ah)

Do you take birth control pills?
¿Toma algún contraceptivo?
('toh-mah ahl-'goon kohn-trah-sehp-'tee-voh)

Allergies

Do you have any allergies?
¿Tiene alergias?
(tee-'eh-neh ah-'lehr-hee-ahs)

Are you allergic to any medicines?
¿Es usted alérgico a algún medicamento?
(ehs oo-'stehd ah-'lehr-hee-co ah ahl-'goon meh-dee-kah-'mehn-toh)

Penicillin
Penicilina
(peh-nee-see-'lee-nah)

Iodine
Yodo
('yoh-doh)

Antibiotics
Antibióticos
(ahn-tee-bee-'oh-tee-kohs)

What kind of reaction do you get?
¿Qué tipo de reacción tiene?
(keh 'tee-poh deh ree-ahk-see-'ohn tee'eh-neh)

Rash
Erupción
(eh-roop-see-'ohn)

Itching
Picazón
(pee-kah-'sohn)

Runny nose
Flujo nasal
('floo-hoh nah-'sahl)

2

Watery eyes
Ojos llorosos
('oh-hos yo-'roh-sohs)

Difficulty breathing
Dificultad para respirar
(dee-fee-kool-'tahd 'pah-rah rehs-pee-'rahr)

Are you allergic to any foods?
¿Es usted alérgico a alguna comida?
(ehs oo-'stehd ah-'lehr-hee-koh ah ahl-'goo-nah koh-'mee-dah)

Eggs
Huevos
('weh-bohs)

Milk
Leche
('leh-cheh)

Gluten
Gluten
('gloo-tehn)

Use of Alternative Medicines

Do you take any over-the-counter medications?
¿Toma usted algún medicamento sin receta?
('toh-mah oo-'stehd ahl-'goon meh-dee-kah-'mehn-toh seen reh-'seh-tah)

Do you take any natural medicines?
¿Toma algún medicamento natural?
('toh-mah ahl-'goon meh-dee-kah-'mehn-toh nah-too-'rahl)

Do you take any natural remedies?
¿Toma algún remedio natural?
('toh-mah ahl-'goon reh-'meh-dee-oh nah-too-'rahl)

Which ones?
¿Cuáles?
('kwahl-ehs)

Chamomile
Manzanilla
(mahn-sah-'nee-yah)

Cinammon tea
Té de canela
(teh deh kah-'neh-lah)

Green tea
Té verde
(teh 'behr-deh)

Vitamins
Vitaminas
(bee-tah-'mee-nahs)

Milk of magnesia
Leche de magnesia
('leh-cheh deh mag-'nehs-ee-ah)

In the Exam Room

3

This chapter outlines the most common questions and occurrences during the subjective data collection process in the examination room. Importantly, this chapter translates the widely used PQRSTU mnemonic to help the nurse organize his or her questions (PQRSTU = Provocative, Quality/Quantity, Region/Radiation, Severity Scale, Timing, Understand Patient's Perception). The most common answers are also listed.

Pain is highly subjective. Varied cultures display it differently. When assessing pain on a Spanish-speaking person, try to find out how it is that she / he usually manifests pain, and how it is that she / he deals with it. You may ask questions such as, *¿Qué hace usualmente cuando tiene dolor?* *(keh 'ah-seh 'oo-swahl-'mehn-teh 'kwahn-doh tee-'eh-neh doh-'lohr)* (What do you usually do when you have pain?). Or you may want to offer words of assurance: *Déjeme saber si tiene dolor* *(deh-'heh-meh sah-'behr see tee-'eh-neh doh-'lohr)* (let me know whether you have pain), or comfort: *Estoy aquí para darle su medicamento para el dolor* *(ehs-'toy ah-'kee 'pah-rah 'dahr-leh soo meh-dee-kah-'mehn-toh 'pah-rah ehl doh-'lohr)* (I am here to give you your pain medication).

Do not assume that a Spanish-speaking patient does not have any pain just because she or he is not saying anything. Ask questions; you will be glad you did.

➤ HISTORY OF PRESENT ILLNESS

Please tell me about your _____.
Por favor, dígame acerca de su _____.
(pohr fah-'bohr, 'dee-gah-meh ah-'sehr-kah deh soo_____)

Headache
Dolor de cabeza
(doh-'lohr deh kah-'beh-sah)

Chest pain
Dolor de pecho
(doh-'lohr deh 'peh-choh)

Fever
Fiebre
(fee-'eh-breh)

Abdominal pain
Dolor abdominal (Dolor de estómago)
(doh-'lohr ahb-doh-mee-'nahl (doh-'lohr deh eh-'stoh-mah-goh))

Blurred vision
Visión borrosa
(bee-see-'ohn boh-'rroh-sah)

Dizziness
Mareo
(mah-'reh-oh)

Leg pain
Dolor de pierna
(doh-'lohr deh pee-'ehr-nah)

Shortness of breath
Sofocamiento (falto de respiración)
(soh-foh-kah-mee-'ehn-toh ('fahl-toh deh rehs-pee-rah-see-'ohn))

3

P: *Provocative*

What causes the pain?
¿Qué le causa el dolor?
(keh leh 'kow-sah ehl doh-'lohr)

Food
Comida (alimentos)
(koh-'mee-dah) (ah-lee-mee-'ehn-tohs)

Breathing deep
Respiraciones profundas
(rehs-pee-rah-see-'ohn-ehs proh-'foon-dahs)

Exercising
Ejercicio
(eh-hehr-'see-see-oh)

What makes the pain worse?
¿Qué le agrava el dolor?
(keh leh ah-'grah-bah ehl doh-'lohr)

Standing
Estar de pie
(eh-'stahr deh pee-'eh)

Bending
Doblarse
(doh-'blahr-seh)

Lying down
Acostarse
(ah-koh-'stahr-seh)

Food
Comida
(koh-'mee-dah)

Walking
Caminar
(kah-mee-'nahr)

Running
Correr
(koh-'rrehr)

What makes the pain better?
¿Qué le mejora el dolor?
(keh leh meh-'hohr-ah ehl doh-'lohr)

Medication
Medicamento
(meh-dee-kah-'mehn-toh)

Rest
Descanso
(dehs-'kahn-soh)

Cold
Frio
('free-oh)

Warmth
Tibio
('tee-bee-oh)

Q: *Quality or Quantity*

Do you have pain?
¿Tiene dolor?
(tee-'eh-neh doh-'lohr)

How does it feel?
¿Cómo se siente?
('koh-moh seh see-'ehn-teh)

Describe your pain.
Describa su dolor.
(dehs-'kree-bah soo doh-'lohr)

Acute?
¿Agudo?
(ah-'goo-doh)

Burning?
¿Le quema?
(leh 'keh-mah)

Comes and goes?
¿Va y viene?
(bah ee bee-'eh-neh)

Does it bother you?
¿Le molesta?
(leh moh-'leh-stah)

R: *Region or Radiation*

Where do you have your pain?
¿Donde tiene el dolor?
('dohn-deh tee-'eh-neh ehl doh-'lohr)

In my head
En la cabeza
(ehn lah kah-'beh-sah)

In my ears
En los oídos
(ehn lohs oh-'ee-dohs)

In my eyes
En los ojos
(ehn lohs 'oh-hohs)

In my mouth
En la boca
(ehn lah 'boh-kah)

In my tooth (teeth)
En el diente (los dientes)
(ehn ehl dee-'ehn-teh) (lohs dee-'ehn-tehs)

In my throat
En la garganta
(ehn lah gahr-'gahn-tah)

In my chest
En el pecho
(ehn ehl 'peh-choh)

In my arms
En los brazos
(ehn lohs 'brah-sohs)

In my hands
En las manos
(ehn lahs 'mah-nohs)

In my fingers
En los dedos
(ehn lohs 'deh-dohs)

In my fingernail
En la uña
(ehn lah 'oon-yah)

In my stomach
En el estómago
(ehn ehl eh-'stoh-mah-goh)

In my womb
En la matriz
(ehn lah mah-'treehs)

In my penis
En el pene
(ehn ehl 'peh-neh)

In my legs
En las piernas
(ehn lahs pee-'ehr-nahs)

In my feet
En los pies
(ehn lohs pee-'ehs)

In my toes
En los dedos de los pies
(ehn lohs 'deh-dohs deh lohs pee-'ehs)

Where does it go?
¿A donde se va el dolor?
(ah 'dohn-deh seh bah ehl doh-'lohr)

To the left arm?
Al brazo izquierdo
(ahl 'brah-soh ees-kee-'ehr-doh)

To the throat
Al cuello / A la garganta
(ahl 'kweh-yoh) (ah lah gahr-'gahn-tah)

To my right side
A mi lado derecho
(ah mee 'lah-doh deh-'reh-choh)

To my left side
A mi lado izquierdo
(ah mee 'lah-doh ees-kee-'ehr-doh)

Below
Para abajo
(pah-rah ah-'bah-hoh)

Above
Para arriba
('pah-rah ah-'rree-bah)

S: *Severity Scale*

If zero means no pain, and ten means the greatest pain you ever had,
Si cero es que no hay dolor, y diez el dolor más fuerte que ha tenido
(see 'seh-roh ehs keh noh ah-ee doh-'lohr, ee 'dee-ehs ehl doh-'lohr
mahs foo-'ehr-teh keh hah teh-'nee-doh)

What number do you give your pain?
¿Qué número le da a su dolor?
(keh 'noo-meh-roh leh dah ah soo doh-'lohr)

How much pain do you have?
¿Cuánto dolor tiene?
('kwahn-toh doh-'lohr tee-'eh-neh)

Little (very little)
Poco (poquito)
('poh-koh (poh-'kee-toh))

Moderate (more or less)
Moderado (más o menos)
(moh-deh-'rah-doh (mahs oh 'meh-nohs))

A lot
Mucho
('moo-choh)

T: *Timing*

When did it first happen?
¿Cuándo le pasó por primera vez?
('kwahn-doh leh pah-'soh pohr pree-'meh-rah behs)

Yesterday
Ayer
(ah-'yehr)

Seven hours ago
Hace siete horas
('ah-she see-'eh-teh 'oh-rahs)

Two days ago
Hace dos días
('ah-seh dohs 'dee-ahs)

Three weeks ago
Hace tres semanas
('ah-seh trehs seh-'mah-nahs)

Four months ago
Hace cuatro meses
('ah-seh 'kwa-troh 'meh-sehs)

A year ago
Hace un año
('ah-seh oon 'ahn-yoh)

In the morning
En la mañana
(ehn lah mahn-'yah-nah)

Yesterday evening
Ayer por la tarde
(ah-'yehr pohr lah 'tahr-deh)

Last night
Anoche
(ah-'noh-cheh)

How long does it last?
¿Por cuánto tiempo dura?
(pohr 'kwahn-toh tee-'ehm-poh 'doo-rah)

About fifteen minutes
Como quince minutos
('koh-moh 'keen-seh mee-'noo-tohs)

About an hour
Como una hora
('koh-moh oo-nah 'oh-rah)

How often does it happen?
¿Con cuál frequencia le pasa?
(kohn kwahl freh-'kwehn-see-ah leh 'pah-sah)

Every time I eat
Cada vez que como
('kah-dah behs keh 'koh-moh)

Every time I go to the *bathroom*
Cada vez que voy al baño
('kah-dah behs keh boy ahl 'bah-nyoh)

Every time I get upset
Cada vez que me enojo
('kah-dah behs keh meh eh-'noh-hoh)

Every time I walk
Cada vez que camino
('kah-dah behs keh kah-'mee-noh)

Every time I bend down
Cada vez que me agacho
('kah-dah behs keh meh ah-'gah-choh)

Every time I stand up
Cada vez que me pongo de pie
('kah-dah behs keh meh 'pohn-goh deh pee-'eh)

When I lie down
Cuando me acuesto
('kwahn-doh meh ah-'kwehs-toh)

When I get up
Cuando me levanto
('kwahn-doh meh leh-'vahn-toh)

U: *Understand Patient's Perception*

What do you think it is?
¿Qué piensa usted que es?
(keh pee-'ehn-sah oo'-stehd keh ehs)

Cancer
Cáncer
('kahn-sehr)

Diabetes
Diabetes
(dee-ah-'beh-tehs)

High blood pressure
Presión alta
(preh-see-'ohn 'ahl-tah)

Gastritis
Gastritis
(gahs-'tree-tees)

Stroke
Embolia
(ehm-'boh-lee-ah)

Tumor
Tumor
(too-'mohr)

I do not know.
No sé.
(noh seh)

Fright
Susto
('suhs-toh)

Rage
Coraje
(koh-'rah-heh)

Witchcraft
Embrujo
(ehm-'broo-hoh)

Evil eye
Mal de ojo
(mahl deh 'oh-hoh)

➤ *PAST MEDICAL HISTORY*

Have you had
¿Ha tenido?
(ah teh-'nee-doh)

Measles?
¿Sarampión?
(sah-rahm-pee-'ohn)

Mumps?
¿Paperas?
(pah-'peh-rahs)

Rubella?
¿Rubéola?
(roo-'beh-oh-lah)

Chicken pox?
¿Varicela?
(bah-ree-'seh-lah)

Scarlet fever?
¿Fiebre Escarlatina?
(fee-'eh-breh ehs-kahr-lah-'tee-nah)

Poliomyelitis?
¿Poliomielitis?
(poh-lee-oh-meh-'lee-tees)

Rheumatic fever?
¿Fiebre Reumática?
(fee-'eh-breh reh-oo-'mah-tee-kah)

Fractures?
¿Fracturas?
(frahk-'too-rahs)

Wounds?
¿Heridas?
(eh-'ree-dahs)

Head contusions?
¿Contusiones en la cabeza?
(kohn-too-see-'ohn-ehs ehn lah kah-'beh-sah)

Burns?
¿Quemaduras?
(keh-mah-'doo-rahs)

Do you have diabetes?
¿Tiene diabetes?
(tee-'eh-neh dee-ah-'beh-tehs)

Hypertension?
¿Presión alta?
(preh-see-'ohn 'ahl-tah)

Heart disease?
¿Enfermedades del corazón?
(ehn-fehr-meh-'dah-dehs dehl koh-rah-'sohn)

Cancer?
¿Cáncer?
('kahn-sehr)

Have you ever been hospitalized?
¿Ha estado alguna vez hospitalizado?
(ah ehs-'tah-doh ahl-'goon-nah behs ohs-pee-tahl-ee-'sah-doh)

Have you ever been in a car accident?
¿Ha estado alguna vez en un accidente de automóvil?
(ah ehs-'tah-doh ahl-'goon-nah behs ehn oon ahk-see-'dehn-teh de ow-toh-'moh-beel)

Have you ever had surgery?
¿Ha tenido alguna cirugía?
(ah teh-'nee-doh ahl-'goon-ah see-roo-'hee-ah)

What kind?
¿Qué tipo?
(keh 'tee-poh)

Appendix
Apéndice
(ah-'pehn-dee-seh)

Stomach
Estómago
(ehs-'toh-mah-goh)

Heart
Corazón
(koh-rah-'sohn)

Spleen
Bazo
('bah-soh)

Hernia
Hernia
('ehr-nee-ah)

Hysterectomy
Histerectomía
(ees-teh-rehk-toh-'mee-ah)

Cesarean section
Sección cesárea
(sehk-see-'ohn seh-'sah-ree-ah)

How many times have you been pregnant?
¿Cuántas veces ha estado embarazada?
('kwahn-tahs 'beh-sehs ha ehs-'tah-doh ehm-bah-rah-'sah-dah)

How many children do you have?

¿Cuántos hijos / hijas tiene?

('kwahn-tohs 'ee-hohs / 'ee-hahs tee-'eh-neh)

Have you ever had an abortion (miscarriage)?

¿Ha tenido alguna vez un aborto (malparto)?

(ah teh-'nee-doh ahl-'goo-nah behs oon ah-'bohr-toh (mahl-'pahr-toh))

Do you have all your immunizations?

¿Tiene todas sus vacunas?

(tee-'eh-neh 'toh-dahs soohs vah-'koo-nahs)

Measles-mumps-rubella

Sarampión-paperas-rubéola

(sah-rahm-pee-'ohn pah-'peh-rahs roo-'beh-oh-lah)

Polio

Polio

('poh-lee-oh)

Diphtheria-tetanus

Difteria-tétano

(deef-'teh-ree-ah / 'teh-tah-noh)

Hepatitis B

Hepatitis B

(ehp-ah-'tee-tees beh)

Pneumococcal vaccine

Vacuna neumocócica

(bah-'koo-nah neh-oohm-oh-'koh-see-kah)

Flu vaccine

Vacuna contra la gripe

(bah-'koo-nah 'kon-trah lah 'gree-peh)

When was your last tetanus vaccine?
¿Cuándo fué su última vacuna contra el tétano?
('kwahn-doh fweh soo 'oohl-tee-mah bah-'koo-nah 'kohn-trah ehl 'teh-tah-noh)

When was your last TB test?
¿Cuándo fué su último examen de tuberculosis?
('kwahn-doh fweh soo 'oohl-tee-moh ehk-'sah-mehn deh too-behr-koo-'loh-seehs)

When was your last flu shot?
¿Cuándo fué su última vacuna contra la gripe?
('kwahn-doh fweh soo 'oohl-tee-mah bah-'koo-nah 'kohn-trah lah 'gree-peh)

When was your last physical exam?
¿Cuándo fue su último examen físico?
('kwahn-doh fweh soo 'oohl-tee-moh ehk-'sah-mehn 'fee-see-koh)

When was your last _____ exam?
¿Cuándo fue su último examen de _____?
('kwahn-doh fweh soo 'oohl-tee-moh ehk-'sah-mehn deh _____)

Eyes
Ojos
('oh-hohs)

Dental
Dental
(dehn-'tahl)

Ears
Oídos
(oh-'ee-dohs)

When was your last _____
¿Cuándo fue su último _____
('kwahn-doh fweh soo 'oohl-tee-moh)

Electrocardiogram
Electrocardiograma
(eh-lehk-troh-kahr-dee-oh-'grah-mah)

Chest X-ray
Rayo X del pecho
('Rah-yoh 'eh-kees dehl 'peh-choh)

3

Review of Systems

4

Before starting a battery of questions during the review of systems, try to gain the client's trust by asking questions that may not necessarily be viewed as related to a physical exam. Once you establish that trust, the client will be more willing to share the answers to questions that are often deemed personal. You may want to start by introducing yourself, and then asking a few questions such as, *¿Cómo está su familia?* (*'koh-moh eh-'stah soo fah-'mee-lee-ah*) (*how is your family?*).

➤ GENERAL

Do you smoke?
¿Fuma usted?
(*'foo-mah oo-'stehd*)

How many packs a day?
¿Cuántos paquetes de cigarillos al día?
(*'kwahn-tohs pah-'keh-tehs deh see-'gah-riyos ahl 'dee-ah*)

For how long have you smoked?
¿Por cuánto tiempo ha fumado?
(*pohr 'kwahn-toh tee-'ehm-poh ah foo-'mah-doh*)

Do you drink alcohol?
¿Toma usted alcohol?
('toh-mah oo-'stehd ahl-koh-'ohl)

How often?
¿Con qué frecuencia?
(kohn keh freh-'kwehn-see-ah)

What kind of liquor?
¿Qué tipo de licor?
(keh 'tee-poh deh lee-'kohr)

When did you quit?
¿Cuándo dejo de tomar?
('kwahn-'doh deh-hoh deh toh-'mahr)

Have you ever taken drugs?
¿Ha tomado drogas alguna vez?
(ah toh-'mah-doh 'droh-gahs ahl-'goo-nah behs)

What kind?
¿Qué tipo?
(keh 'tee-poh)

Marijuana
Marihuana
(mah-ree-'wah-nah)

Cocaine
Cocaina
(koh-kah-'ee-nah)

Heroin
Heroina
(eh-roh-'ee-nah)

Do you exercise?
¿Hace ejercicio?
('ah-seh eh-hehr-'see-see-oh)

What type of exercise do you do?
¿Qué tipo de ejercicio hace?
(keh 'tee-poh deh eh-hehr-'see-see-oh 'ah-seh)

Walk
Caminar
(kah-mee-'nahr)

Run
Correr
(koh-'rrehr)

Swim
Nadar
(nah-'dahr)

Weight lifting
Levantar pesas
(leh-vahn-'tahr 'peh-sahs)

Yoga
Yoga
('yoh-gah)

➤ *HEENT*

Head
Cabeza
(kah-'beh-sah)

Eyes
Ojos
('oh-hohs)

Ears
Oídos
(oh-'ee-dohs)

Nose
Nariz
(nah-'rees)

Throat
Garganta
(gahr-'gahn-tah)

Head

Have you had any headaches lately?
¿Ha tenido dolores de cabeza últimamente?
(ah teh-'nee-doh doh-'loh-rehs deh kah-'beh-sah 'oohl-tee-mah-mehn-teh)

Where do you feel it?
¿Dónde lo siente?
('dohn-deh loh see-'ehn-teh)

Behind your eyes?
¿Detrás de los ojos?
(deh-'trahs deh lohs 'oh-hohs)

On the left side?
¿En el lado izquierdo?
(ehn ehl 'lah-doh ees-kee-'ehr-doh)

On the right side?

¿En el lado derecho?

(ehn ehl 'lah-doh deh-'reh-choh)

On the back of your head?

¿Detrás de su cabeza?

(deh-'trahs deh soo kah-'beh-sah)

All over?

¿Por todos lados?

(pohr 'toh-dohs 'lah-dohs)

Is it mild, moderate, or severe?

¿Es mínimo, moderado, o severo?

(ehs 'mee-nee-moh, moh-deh-'rah-doh, oh seh-'beh-roh)

What time of the day does it occur?

¿A qué horas del día ocurre?

(ah keh 'oh-rahs dehl 'dee-ah oh-'koo-reh)

How long does it last?

¿Por cuánto tiempo dura?

(pohr 'kwahn-toh tee-'ehm-poh 'doo-rah)

What provokes the pain?

¿Qué provoca el dolor?

(keh proh-'boh-kah ehl doh-'lohr)

Is there nausea or vomiting?

¿Tiene nausea o vómito?

(tee-'eh-neh 'now-seh-ah oh 'boh-mee-toh)

What makes it worse?

¿Qué lo empeora?

(keh loh ehm-peh-'ohr-ah)

Coughing, movement, straining, exercise?
¿Tos, moverse, esforsarze, ejercicio?
(tohs, moh-'behr-seh, ehs-fohr-'sahr-seh, eh-hehr-'see-see-oh)

Any head injury or blow to your head?
¿Ha tenido alguna herida en la cabeza?
(ah teh-'nee-doh ahl-'goo-nah eh-'ree-dah ehn lah kah-'beh-sah)

Any blackouts?
¿Algún desmayo?
(ahl-'goon dehs-'mah-yoh)

Seizures?
¿Convulsiones?
(kohn-buhl-see-'ohn-ehs)

Any dizziness?
¿Mareos?
(mah-'reh-ohs)

Any neck pain?
¿Dolor del cuello?
(doh-'lohr dehl 'kweh-yoh)

Any difficulty swallowing?
¿Dificultad para tragar?
(dee-fee-kool-'tahd pah-rah trah-'gahr)

Have you ever had any thyroid problems?
¿Ha tenido problemas con la tiroide?
(ah teh-'nee-doh proh-'bleh-mahs kohn lah tee-'roh-ee-deh)

Eyes

Ojos
('oh-hohs)

Have you had any difficulty seeing?
¿Ha tenido problemas con la vista?
(ah teh-'nee-doh proh-'bleh-mahs kohn lah 'bees-tah)

Any blurring
¿Visión borrosa?
(bee-see-'ohn boh-'roh-sah)

Which eye?
¿Cuál ojo?
(kwahl 'oh-hoh)

Right
Derecho
(deh-'reh-choh)

Left
Izquierdo
(ees-kee-'ehr-doh)

Both
Los dos
(lohs dohs)

Does it come and go?
¿Va y viene?
(bah ee bee-'eh-neh)

Is it constant?
¿Es constante?
(ehs kohn-'stahn-teh)

Any difficulty seeing at night?
¿Tiene dificultad de ver en la noche?
(tee-'eh-neh dee-fee-kool-'tahd deh behr ehn lah 'noh-cheh)

Any pain?
¿Algún dolor?
(ahl-'goon doh-'lohr)

Any history of crossed eyes?
¿Ha tenido estrabismo?
(ah teh-'nee-doh eh-strah-'bees-moh)

Any redness or swelling?
¿Ha tenido los ojos rojos o hinchados?
(ah teh-'nee-doh lohs 'oh-hohs 'roh-hohs oh een-'chah-dohs)

Any history of injury or surgery to the eyes?
¿Ha tenido alguna herida o cirugia en los ojos?
(ah teh-'nee-doh ahl-'goo-nah eh-'ree-dah o see-roo-'hee-ah en lohs 'oh-hohs)

Have you ever had glaucoma?
¿Ha tenido alguna vez glaucoma?
(ah teh-'nee-doh ahl-'goo-nah behs glahw-'koh-mah)

Have you ever been tested for glaucoma?
¿Le han hecho el examen del glaucoma?
(leh ahn 'eh-choh ehl ehk-'sah-mehn dehl glahw-'koh-mah)

Do you use glasses?
¿Usa lentes?

('oo-sah 'lehn-tehs)

When did you last visit the eye doctor?
¿Cuándo fue la última vez que vio al doctor de los ojos?
('kwahn-doh fweh lah 'oohl-tee-mah behs keh bee-'oh ahl dohk-'tohr deh lohs 'oh-hohs)

Ears

Oídos
(oh-'ee-dohs)

Have you had any earache?
¿Tiene dolor de oídos?
(tee-'eh-neh doh-'lohr deh oh-'ee-dohs)

Any history of constant ear infections?
¿Ha tenido infecciones constantes de los oídos?
(ah teh-'nee-doh een-fehk-see-'oh-nehs kohn-'stahn-tehs deh lohs oh-'ee-dohs)

Any discharge from your ears?
¿Alguna supuración de los oídos?
(ahl-'goo-nah soo-poo-rah-see-'ohn deh lohs oh-'ee-dohs)

Have you had any trouble hearing?
¿Ha tenido alguna vez problema con oir?
(ah teh-'nee-doh ahl-'goon-ah behs proh-'bleh-mah kohn oh-'eer)

Have you been exposed to a great deal of noise?
¿Ha estado expuesto a mucho ruido?
(ah eh-'stah-doh ehk-spu-'ehs-toh ah 'moo-choh roo-'ee-doh)

Ever felt ringing, crackling, or buzzing in your ears?
¿Alguna vez ha sentido un zumbido, ruido, o tintineo en los oídos?
(ahl-'goon-ah behs ah sehn-'tee-doh oon zoom-'bee-doh, roo-'ee-doh, oh teen-tee-'neh-oh ehn lohs oh-'ee-dohs)

Ever felt vertigo or dizziness?
¿Ha sentido vertigo o mareos alguna vez?
(ah sehn-'tee-doh behr-'tee-goh oh mah-'reh-ohs ahl-'goo-nah behs)

How do you clean your ears?
¿Cómo se limpia los oídos?
('koh-moh seh 'leehm-pee-ah lohs oh-'ee-dohs)

Nose, Mouth, and Throat

Nariz, Boca, y Garganta
(nah-'rees, 'boh-kah, ee garh-'gahn-tah)

Do you have a runny nose?
¿Le gotea la nariz?
(leh 'goh-teh-ah lah nah-'rees)

Clear?
¿Claro?
('klah-roh)

Bloody?
¿Con sangre?
(kohn 'sahn-greh)

Purulent?
¿Purulento?
(poo-roo-'lehn-toh)

Any nosebleeds?
¿Le sangra la nariz?
(leh 'sahn-grah lah nah-'rees)

Can you smell?
¿Puede oler?
('pweh-deh oh-'lehr)

Any sores in your mouth?
¿Tiene alguna llaga en la boca?
(tee-'eh-neh ahl-'goon-nah 'yah-gah ehn lah 'boh-kah)

Do you have a sore throat?
¿Le duele la garganta?
(leh 'dweh-leh lah gahr-'gahn-tah)

Any bleeding gums?
¿Le sangran las encías?
(leh 'sahn-grahn lahs ehn-'see-ahs)

Do you have a toothache?
¿Tiene dolor de diente?
(tee-'eh-neh doh-'lohr deh dee-'ehn-teh)

Are your teeth sensitive to cold? Hot?
¿Son sensitivos sus dientes a lo frio, lo caliente?
(sohn sehn-see-'tee-bohs soos dee-'ehn-tehs ah loh 'free-oh, loh kah-lee-'ehn-teh)

Any difficulty swallowing?
¿Tiene dificultad para tragar?
(tee-'eh-neh dee-fee-kool-'tahd 'pah-rah trah-'gahr)

Can you taste?
¿Puede saborear?
('pweh-deh sah-boh-ree-'ahr)

➤ RESPIRATORY

Do you have a cough?
¿Tiene tos?
(tee-'eh-neh tohs)

When did it start?
¿Cuándo empezó?
('kwahn-doh ehm-peh-'soh)

How long have you had it?
¿Por cuánto tiempo lo ha tenido?
(pohr 'kwahn-toh tee-'ehm-poh loh ah teh-'nee-doh)

How often do you cough?
¿Con qué frecuencia tose?
(kohn keh freh-kwehn-see-ah 'toh-seh)

Are you coughing up any phlegm?
¿Está tociendo alguna flema?
(eh-'stah toh-see-'ehn-doh ahl-'goo-nah 'fleh-mah)

Do you feel short of breath?
¿Le falta la respiración?
(leh 'fahl-tah lah rehs-pee-rah-see-'ohn)

Have you had any problems breathing in the past?
¿Ha tenido algún problema con la respiración en el pasado?
(ah teh-'nee-doh ahl-'goon proh-'bleh-mah kohn lah rehs-pee-rah-see-'ohn ehn ehl pah-'sah-doh)

Do you have asthma?
¿Tiene asma?
(tee-'eh-neh 'ahs-mah)

Emphysema?
¿Enfisema?
(ehn-fee-'seh-mah)

Pneumonia?
¿Neumonía?
(neh-oo-moh-'nee-ah)

Lung cancer?
¿Cancer del pulmón?
('kahn-sehr dehl pool-'mohn)

➤ *CARDIOVASCULAR*

Do you have any chest pain?
¿Tiene dolor del pecho?
(tee-'eh-neh doh-'lohr dehl 'peh-choh)

Have you ever had this pain before?
¿Ha tenido este dolor alguna vez antes?
(ah teh-'nee-doh 'eh-steh doh-'lohr ahl-'goo-nah behs 'ahn-tehs)

Where did the pain start?
¿Dónde empezó el dolor?
('dohn-deh ehm-peh-soh' ehl doh-'lohr)

Do you have it anywhere else?
¿Lo tiene en algún otro lugar?
(loh tee-'eh-neh ehn ahl-'goon 'oh-troh loo-'gahr)

Does the pain gets worse with activity?
¿Se empeora el dolor con la actividad?
(seh ehm-peh-'oh-rah ehl doh-'lohr kohn lah ahk-tee-bee-'dahd)

Deep breathing?
¿Con la respiración profunda?
(kohn lah rehs-pee-rah-see-'ohn proh-'foon-dah)

Changing position?
¿Cambiando de posición?
(kahm-bee-'ahn-doh deh poh-see-see-'ohn)

4

Does it get better with nitroglycerin?
¿Se mejora con nitroglicerina?
(seh meh-'hoh-rah kohn nee-troh-glee-seh-'ree-nah)

How many pills do you take?
¿Cuántas pastillas toma usted?
('kwahn-tahs pahs-'tee-yahs 'toh-mah oo-'stehd)

Do you have any shortness of breath?
¿Le falta la respiración?
(leh 'fahl-tah lah rehs-pee-rah-see-'ohn)

Do you get tired easily?
¿Se cansa pronto?
(seh 'kahn-sah 'prohn-toh)

Are your legs / feet swollen?
¿Se le hinchan las piernas / los pies?
(seh leh 'eehn-chahn lahs pee-'ehr-nahs / lohs pee-'ehs)

Have you had high blood pressure?
¿Ha tenido presión alta?
(ah teh-'nee-doh preh-see-'ohn 'ahl-tah)

High cholesterol?
¿Colesterol alto?
(kohl-ehs-teh-'rohl 'ahl-toh)

Rheumatic fever?
¿Fiebre reumática?
(fee-'eh-breh reh-oo-'mah-tee-kah)

Have you ever had heart surgery?
¿Ha tenido cirugía del corazón?
(ah teh-'nee-doh see-roo-'hee-ah dehl koh-rah-'sohn)

When was your last electrocardiogram?
¿Cuándo fue su último electrocardiograma?
('kwahn-doh fweh soo 'ool-tee-moh eh-lehk-troh-kahr-dee-oh-'grah-mah)

What heart medications do you take?
¿Qué medicamentos toma?
(keh meh-dee-kah-'mehn-tohs 'toh-mah)

Does anyone in your family have heart trouble?
¿Alguien en su familia tiene problemas con el corazón?
('ahl-gee-ehn ehn soo fah-'mee-lee-ah tee-'eh-neh proh-'bleh-mahs kohn ehl koh-rah-'sohn)

➤ *GASTROINTESTINAL*

Has your appetite changed?
¿Ha cambiado su apetito?
(ah kahm-bee-'ah-doh soo ah-peh-'tee-toh)

Have you lost any weight?
¿Ha perdido peso?
(ah pehr-'dee-doh 'peh-soh)

Have you gained any weight?
¿Ha ganado peso?
(ah gah-'nah-doh 'peh-soh)

Have you been on a diet?
¿Está a dieta?
(eh-'stah ah dee'-eh-tah)

Have you had any abdominal pain?
¿Tiene dolor del estómago?
(tee-'eh-neh doh-'lohr dehl ehs-'toh-mah-goh)

Where?
¿Dónde?
('dohn-deh)

Have you had any nausea or vomiting?
¿Ha tenido nausea o vómito?
(ah teh-'nee-doh 'nahw-see-ah oh 'boh-mee-toh)

Any blood in your vomit?
¿Tiene sangre en el vómito?
(tee-'eh-neh 'sahn-greh ehn ehl 'boh-mee-toh)

Any blood in your stool?
¿Tiene sangre en el excremento?
(tee-'eh-neh 'sahn-greh ehn ehl ehks-kreh-mehn-toh)

Have you ever had any gastrointestinal problems?
¿Ha tenido problemas gastro-intestinales?
(ah teh-'nee-doh proh-'bleh-mahs gahs-troh-een-tehs-tee-'nahl-ehs)

Diarrhea?
¿Diarrea?
(dee-ah-'rreh-ah)

Constipation?
¿Estreñido?
(ehs-treh-'nyee-doh)

Ulcer?
¿Úlcera?
('ool-seh-rah)

Gallbladder stones?
¿Piedras en la vesícula?
(pee-'eh-drahs ehn lah beh-'see-koo-lah)

Surgeries?
¿Cirugías?
(see-roo-'hee-ahs)

Appendicitis?
¿Apendicitis?
(ah-pehn-dee-'see-tees)

Colitis?
¿Colitis?
(koh-'lee-tees)

Hernia?
¿Hernia?
('ehr-nee-ah)

Hepatitis?
¿Hepatitis?
(ehp-ah-'tee-tees)

➤ *GENITOURINARY*

Men

Are you urinating more often than usual?
¿Orina más de lo usual?
(oh-'ree-nah mahs deh loh oo-soo-'ahl)

Any pain or burning with urinating?
¿Tiene dolor o le arde cuando orina?
(tee-'eh-neh doh-'lohr oh leh 'ahr-deh 'kwahn-doh oh-'ree-nah)

Any trouble starting the urine stream?
¿Tiene problemas al empezar a orinar?
(tee-'eh-neh proh-'bleh-mahs ahl ehm-peh-'sahr ah oh-ree-'nahr)

What color is your urine?
¿Qué color es su orina?
(keh koh-'lohr ehs soo oh-'ree-nah)

Clear?
¿Clara?
('klah-rah)

Cloudy?
¿Turbia?
('tour-bee-ah)

Foul-smelling?
¿De mal olor?
(deh mahl oh-'lohr)

Bloody?
¿Con sangre?
(kohn 'sahn-greh)

Any discharge?
¿Algún desecho?
(ahl-'goon dehs-'eh-choh)

Women

When was your last menstrual period?
¿Cuándo fue su último periodo?
('kwahn-doh fweh soo 'ool-tee-moh peh-ree-'oh-doh)

How often is your period?
¿Con qué frecuencia es su periodo?
(kohn keh freh-'kwehn-see-ah ehs soo peh-ree-'oh-doh)

How many days does your period last?
¿Cuántos días dura su periodo?
('kwahn-tohs 'dee-ahs 'doo-rah soo pehr-ree-'oh-doh)

Any pain or cramps before or during your period?
¿Algún dolor o torceduras antes o durante su periodo?
(ahl-'goon doh-'lohr oh tohr-seh-'doo-rahs 'ahn-tehs oh doo-'rahn-teh soo peh-ree-'oh-doh)

Any unusual vaginal discharge?
¿Algún desecho no usual?
(ahl-'goon dehs-'eh-choh noh oo-soo-'ahl)

What is it like?
¿Cómo es?
('koh-moh ehs)

White?
¿Blanco?
('blahn-koh)

Yellowish?
¿Amarillento?
(ah-mah-ree-'yehn-toh)

Greenish?
¿Verdoso?
(behr-'doh-soh)

Curdlike?
¿Cuajo?
('kwah-hoh)

When was your last papanicolaou smear?
¿Cuándo fue su último papanicolaou?
('kwahn-doh fweh soo 'ool-tee-moh pah-pah-nee-koh-'lah-oh)

Do you use contraceptives?
¿Usa contraceptivos?
('oo-sah kohn-trah-sehp-'tee-bohs)

➤ *MUSCULOSKELETAL*

Any pain in your joints?
¿Algún dolor en sus coyunturas?
(ahl-'goon doh-'lohr ehn soos koh-yoon-'too-rahs)

Shoulder?
¿Hombro?
('ohm-broh)

Elbow?
¿Codo?
('koh-doh)

Wrist?
¿Muñeca?
(moo-'nyeh-kah)

Fingers?
¿Dedos?
('deh-dohs)

Hip?
¿Cadera?
(kah-'deh-rah)

Knee?
¿Rodilla?
(rroh-'dee-yah)

Ankle?
¿Tobillo?
(toh-'bee-yoh)

Any swelling or redness in your joints?
¿Alguna inflamación o enrojecimiento en las coyunturas?
(ahl-'goo-nah een-flah-mah-see-'ohn oh ehn-roh-heh-see-mee-'ehn-toh ehn lahs koh-yoon-'too-rahs)

Any difficulty moving your joints?
¿Alguna dificultad para mover las coyunturas?
(ahl-'goo-nah dee-fee-kool-'tahd 'pah-rah moh-'behr lahs koh-yoon-'too-rahs)

Any weakness in your muscles?
¿Alguna debilidad en sus músculos?
(ahl-'goo-nah deh-bee-lee-'dahd ehn soos 'moos-koo-lohs)

Any accidents or fractures?
¿Algún accidente o fractura?
(ahl-'goon ahk-see-'dehn-teh oh frahk-'too-rah)

Have you ever had a fracture of the _____?
¿Ha tenido alguna fractura de _____?
(ah teh-'nee-doh ahl-'goo-nah frahk-'too-rah deh)

Neck?
¿Cuello?
('kweh-yoh)

Back?
¿Espalda?
(ehs-'pahl-dah)

Arm?
¿Brazo?
('brah-soh)

Forearm?
¿Antebrazo?
(ahn-teh-'brah-soh)

Hand?
¿Mano?
(ʹmah-noh)

Leg?
¿Pierna?
(pee-ʹehr-nah)

Feet?
¿Pies?
(pee-ʹehs)

Toes?
¿Dedos de los pies?
(ʹdeh-dohs deh lohs pee-ʹehs)

➤ *NEUROLOGIC*

Any shakes or tremors?
¿Tiene temblores o estremecimientos?
(tee-ʹeh-neh tehm-ʹblohr-ehs oh ehs-treh-meh-see-mee-ʹehn-tohs)

Any weakness?
¿Alguna debilidad?
(ahl-ʹgoon-nah deh-bee-lee-ʹdahd)

Any problems with coordination?
¿Algún problema con la coordinación?
(ahl-ʹgoon proh-ʹbleh-mah kohn lah kohr-dee-nah-see-ʹohn)

Any numbness or tingling?
¿Algún entumecimiento u hormigueo?
(ahl-ʹgoon ehn-too-meh-see-mee-ʹehn-toh uh ohr-mee-ʹgeh-oh)

Any difficulty speaking?
¿Alguna dificultad para hablar?
(ahl-'goo-nah dee-fee-kool-'tahd 'pah-rah ah-'blahr)

Have you had a stroke?
¿Ha tenido una embolia?
(ah teh-'nee-doh 'oo-nah ehm-'boh-lee-ah)

Spinal cord injury?
¿Herida en la médula espinal?
(eh-'ree-dah ehn lah 'meh-doo-lah ehs-'pee-nahl)

Meningitis?
¿Meningitis?
(meh-neen-'hee-tees)

Encephalitis?
¿Encefalitis?
(ehn-seh-fah-'lee-tees)

Congenital defect?
¿Defecto congenital?
(deh-'fehk-toh kohn-heh-nee-'tahl)

Alcoholism?
¿Alcoholismo?
(ahl-koh-ohl-'ees-moh)

Hematologic

Have you ever had anemia?
¿Ha tenido anemia alguna vez?
(ah teh-'nee-doh ah-'neh-mee-ah ahl-'goo-nah behs)

Do you bruise easily?
¿Se moretea (malluga) fácilmente?
(seh moh-reh-'teh-ah (mah-'yoo-gah) 'fah-seel-mehn-teh)

Do you bleed easily?
¿Sangra fácilmente?
('sahn-grah 'fah-seel-mehn-teh)

Do you bleed for a long time?
¿Sangra por mucho tiempo?
('sahn-grah pohr 'moo-choh tee-'ehm-poh)

Do you bleed a lot?
¿Sangra mucho?
('sahn-grah 'moo-choh)

Have you ever had a blood transfusion?
¿Ha tenido alguna vez una transfusión de sangre?
(ah teh-'nee-doh ahl-'goo-nah behs 'oo-nah trahns-foo-see-'ohn deh 'sahn-greh)

Do you have frequent *nosebleeds?*
¿Le sangra la nariz frecuentemente?
(leh 'sahn-grah lah nah-'rees freh-kwehn-teh-'mehn-teh)

Do your gums bleed easily?
¿Le sangran las encías fácilmente?
(leh 'sahn-grahn lahs' ehn-see-ahs 'fah-seel-mehn-teh)

Have you had a fever lately?
¿Ha tenido fiebre últimamente?
(ah teh-'nee-doh fee-'eh-breh 'ool-tee-mah-mehn-teh)

Do you tire easily?
¿Se cansa fácilmente?
(seh 'kahn-sah 'fah-seel-mehn-teh)

Do you get short of breath easily?
¿Se agita fácilmente?
(seh ah-'hee-tah 'fah-seel-mehn-teh)

Do you ever have palpitations?
¿Tiene palpitaciones?
(tee-'eh-neh pahl-pee-tah-see-'ohn-ehs)

Do you have leg pain frequently?
¿Le duelen las piernas frecuentemente?
(leh 'dweh-lehn lahs pee-'ehr-nahs freh-kwehn-teh-'mehn-teh)

Do you have frequent
Tiene frecuentemente
(tee-'eh-neh freh-kwehn-teh-'mehn-teh)

Headaches?
¿Dolores de cabeza?
(doh-'loh-rehs deh kah-'beh-sah)

Dizziness?
¿Mareos?
(mah-'reh-ohs)

Nausea?
¿Nausea?
('now-see-ah)

Intolerance to cold?
¿Intolerancia al frío?
(een-toh-leh'-rahn-seeahl 'free-oh)

Loss of libido?
¿Falta de apetito sexual?
('fahl-tah deh ah-peh-'tee-toh sex-soo-'ahl)

Impotence?
¿Impotencia?
(eem-poh-'tehn-see-ah)

Do you take
Toma usted
('toh-mah oo-'stehd)

Aspirin?
¿Aspirina?
(ahs-pee-'ree-nah)

Coumadin?
¿Cumadina?
(koo-mah-'dee-nah)

Blood thinners?
¿Adelgazadores de sangre?
(ah-dehl-gah-sah-'doh-rehs deh 'sahn-greh)

➤ *ENDOCRINE*

Have you ever had diabetes?
¿Ha tenido diabetes?
(ah teh-'nee-doh dee-ah-'beh-tehs)

Have you ever had problems with
Ha tenido problemas con
(ah teh-'nee-doh proh-'bleh-mahs kohn)

Thyroid?
¿Tiroides?
(tee-'roh-ee-dehs)

Pancreas?
¿Páncreas?
('pahn-kreh-ahs)

Female hormones?
¿Hormonas femeninas?
(ohr-'moh-nahs feh-meh-'nee-nahs)

Estrogen?
¿Estrógeno?
(ehs-'troh-heh-noh)

Male hormones?
¿Hormonas masculinas?
(ohr-'moh-nahs mahs-koo-'lee-nahs)

Testosterone?
¿Testosterona?
(tehs-tohs-tehr-'oh-nah)

Any changes to the color of your skin?
¿Le ha cambiado el color de su piel?
(leh ah kahm-bee-'ah-doh ehl koh-'lohr deh soo pee-'ehl)

How often do you go to the bathroom to void?
¿Con cuánta frequencia va al baño a orinar?
(kohn 'kwahn-tah freh-'kwehn-see-ah bah ahl 'bah-nyoh ah oh-ree-'nahr)

Are you thirsty frequently?
¿Tiene sed frecuentemente?
(tee-'eh-neh sehd freh-kwehn-teh-'mehn-teh)

Are you hungry frequently?
¿Tiene hambre frecuentemente?
(tee-'eh-neh 'ahm-breh freh-kwehn-teh-'mehn-teh)

Do you feel cold most of the time?
¿Se siente con frío la mayoria del tiempo?
(seh see-'ehn-teh kohn 'free-oh lah mah-yoh-'ree-ah dehl tee-'ehm-poh)

Do you sweat a lot?
¿Suda mucho?
('soo-dah 'moo-choh)

Very little?
¿Muy poco?
('moo-ee 'poh-koh)

➤ *MENTAL STATUS*

Orientation

What's your name?
¿Cómo se llama?
('koh-moh seh 'yah-mah)

What's your husband/wife's name?
¿Cómo se llama su esposo/esposa?
('koh-moh se 'yah-mah soo ehs-'poh-soh / ehs-'poh-sah)

Do you know what day is today?
¿Sabe qué día es hoy?
('sah-beh keh 'dee-ah ehs 'oh-ee)

What month is it?
¿Qué mes es?
(keh mehs ehs)

What year is it?
¿Qué año es?
(keh 'ahn-yoh ehs)

Who is the President of the United States?
¿Quién es el presidente de los Estados Unidos?
(kee-'ehn ehs ehl preh-see-'dehn-teh deh lohs eh-'stah-dohs oo-'nee-dohs)

What did you have for breakfast this morning?
¿Qué desayuno tuvo esta mañana?
(keh dehs-ah-'yoo-noh 'too-boh 'ehs-tahmahn-'ya-nah)

What year did you marry?
¿En qué año se casó?
(ehn keh 'ahn-yoh seh kah-'soh)

What are the names of your children?
¿Cómo se llaman sus hijos / hijas?
('koh-moh seh 'ya-mahn soos 'ee-hohs / 'ee-hahs)

Psychiatric

Do you feel anxious most of the time?
¿Se siente nervioso la mayoría del tiempo?
(seh see-'ehn-teh nehr-bee-'oh-soh lah ma-yoh-'ree-ah dehl tee-'ehm-poh)

Do you feel sad most of the time?
¿Se siente triste la mayoría del tiempo?
(seh see-'ehn-teh 'trees-teh lah mah-yoh-'ree-ah dehl tee-'ehm-poh)

What makes you cry?
¿Qué le hace llorar?
(keh leh 'ah-seh 'yoh-rahr)

What makes you happy?
¿Qué le hace feliz?
(keh leh 'ah-seh feh-'lees)

Have you ever had a psychiatric illness?
¿Ha tenido alguna enfermedad siquiátrica?
(ah teh-'nee-doh ahl-'goo-nah ehn-fehr-meh-'dahd see-kee-'ah-tree-kah)

Have you ever been depressed?
¿Ha estado alguna vez deprimido(a)?
(ah ehs-'tah-doh ahl-'goo-nah behs deh-pree-'mee-doh / deh-pree-'mee-dah)

Do you cry easily?
¿Llora fácilmente?
('yo-rah 'fah-seel-mehn-teh)

Do you cry for no reason?
¿Llora sin razón?
('yo-rah seen rah-'sohn)

Do you hear voices?
¿Oye voces?
('oh-yeh 'boh-sehs)

Do you see things?
¿Ve cosas?
(beh 'koh-sahs)

Do you think someone is following you?
¿Piensa que alguien la sigue?
(pee-'ehn-sah keh 'ahl-gee-ehn lah 'see-geh)

Have you ever thought about killing yourself?
¿Ha pensado en matarse alguna vez?
(ah pehn-'sah-doh ehn mah-'tahr-seh ahl-'goo-nah behs)

How?
¿Cómo?
('koh-moh)

Gun?
¿Pistola?
(pee-'stoh-lah)

Knife?
¿Cuchillo?
(koo-'chee-yoh)

Poison?
¿Veneno?
(beh-'neh-noh)

Drowning?
¿Ahogándose?
(ah-oh-'gahn-doh-seh)

Hanging?
¿Colgándose?
(kohl-'gahn-doh-seh)

Do you have a gun?
¿Tiene una pistola?
(tee-'eh-neh 'oo-nah pee'-stoh-lah)

Do you have a knife?
¿Tiene un cuchillo?
(tee-'eh-neh oon koo-'chee-yoh)

Do you have poison in your house?
¿Tiene veneno en su casa?
(tee'-eh-neh beh-'neh-noh ehn soo 'kah-sah)

Have you ever been diagnosed as schizophrenic?
¿Le han diagnosticado alguna vez como esquizofrénico?
(leh ahn dee-ahg-nohs-tee-'kah-doh ahl-'goo-nah behs 'koh-moh ehs-kee-soh-'freh-nee-koh)

Bipolar?
¿Bipolar?
(bee-poh-'lahr)

Obsessive compulsive?
¿Obsesivo compulsivo?
(ohb-seh-'see-boh kohm-pool-'see-boh)

Have you ever been afraid of
Ha tenido alguna vez temor de
(ah teh-'nee-doh ahl-'goo-nah behs teh-'mohr deh)

Being with people?
¿Estar con gente?
(eh-'stahr kohn 'hen-teh)

Being in open spaces?
¿Estar en lugares abiertos?
(eh-'stahr ehn loo-'gahr-ehs ah-bee-'ehr-tohs)

Diagnostic Tests

5

Tests may be stressful to many clients due to the uncertainty of results, as well as the elapsed period of time between collection of data or blood and the actual finding out of the results. Think about how patients who have had an HIV test done feel when they have to wait for the results. The same applies for CT scans, MRIs, X-rays, or blood work. In addition, the monolingual Spanish-speaking patient may not understand the healthcare provider's explanation of the results or may be afraid of not understanding. For situations like these, the healthcare provider may assist the client by providing a few options. For example, ***Voy a llamar a un intérprete*** *(boy ah yah-'mahr ah oon een-'tehr-preh-teh) (I am going to call an interpreter)* or, ***Los resultados de su examen son normales*** *(lohs reh-sool-'tah-dohs deh soo ehk-'sah-mehn sohn nohr-'mahl-ehs) (Your exam results are normal)*. Offering options and being sensitive to the client's potential fears is a necessary step to providing culturally competent nursing care.

➤ *LABORATORY TESTS*

The doctor has ordered some lab tests.
El doctor ha ordenado algunos examenes de laboratorio.
(ehl dohk-'tohr ah ohr-deh-'nah-doh ahl-'goo-nohs ehk-'sah-mehn-ehs deh lah-boh-rah-'toh-ree-oh)

To check your liver
Para examinar su hígado
('pah-rah ehk-sahm-ee-'nahr soo 'ee-gah-doh)

To check your kidneys
Para examinar sus riñones
('pah-rah ehk-sahm-ee-'nahr soos ree-'nyohn-ehs)

To check your heart
Para examinar su corazón
('pah-rah ehk-sahm-ee-'nahr soo koh-rah-'sohn)

To check your thyroid
Para examinar sus tiroides
('pah-rah ehk-sahm-ee-'nahr soos tee-'roh-ee-dehs)

To check your stomach
Para examinar su estómago
('pah-rah ehk-sahm-ee-'nahr soo ehs-'toh-mah-goh)

I am going to draw some blood.
Voy a sacarle sangre.
(boy ah sah-'kahr-leh 'sahn-gre)

I will need a urine sample.
Necesito una muestra de orina.
(neh-seh-'see-toh 'oo-nah 'mwehs-trah deh oo-'ree-nah)

I will need a stool sample.

Necesito una muestra de excremento.

(neh-seh-'see-toh 'oo-nah 'mwehs-trah deh ehks-kreh-'mehn-toh)

I will need a sputum sample.

Necesito una muestra de flema (esputo).

(neh-seh-'see-toh oo-nah 'mweh-strah deh 'fleh-mah)(ehs-'poo-toh)

You will need to fast from midnight until

Necesita ayunar desde la medianoche hasta

(neh-seh-'see-tah ah-yoo-'nahr 'dehs-deh lah meh-dee-ah-'noh-cheh 'ahs-tah)

The blood is drawn.

Que le saquen la sangre.

(keh leh 'sah-kehn lah 'sahn-gre)

The test is done.

Que el examen se termine.

(keh ehl ehk-'sah-mehn seh tehr-'mee-neh)

Do not eat or drink anything after midnight.

No coma ni beba nada después de la medianoche.

(noh 'koh-mah nee 'beh-bah 'nah-dah dehs-'pwehs deh lah meh-dee-ah-'noh-cheh)

You need to collect your urine for 24 hours.

Va a necesitar recolectar su orina por 24 horas.

(bah ah neh-seh-see-'tahr reh-koh-lehk-'tahr soo oh-'ree-nah pohr beh-'een-teh ee 'kwah-troh 'oh-rahs)

Starting with your first voiding.

Empezando con la primera orina.

(ehm-peh-'sahn-doh kohn lah pree-'meh-rah oh-'ree-nah)

In the morning
En la mañana
(ehn lah mahn-'yah-nah)

Bring three samples of stool
Traiga tres muestras de excremento
('trah-ee-gah trehs 'mwehs-trahs deh ehks-kreh-'mehn-toh)

Taken on three different days
Tomadas en tres días distintos
(toh-'mah-dahs ehn trehs 'dee-ahs dees-'teen-tohs)

Common Laboratory Tests

Complete blood count (CBC)
Conteo General de Glóbulos
(kohn-'teh-oh heh-neh-'rahl deh 'gloh-boo-lohs)

Chemistry panel
Panel Químico
(pah-'nehl 'kee-mee-koh)

Cardiac enzymes
Enzimas cardiacas
(ehn-'see-mahs kahr-dee-'ah-kahs)

Liver enzymes
Enzimas del hígado
(ehn-'see-mahs dehl 'ee-gah-doh)

HIV
VIH (Virus de inmuno-deficiencia humana)
(beh ee'ah-cheh) ('bee-roos deh een-'moo-noh deh-fee-see-'ehn-see-ah oo-'mah-nah)

Cholesterol
Colesterol
(koh-lehs-teh-'rohl)

H. pylori
H. pilori
('ah-cheh pee-'loh-ree)

➤ *IMAGING TESTS*

The doctor wants you to have a CT (computed tomography) scan
El doctor quiere hacer una técnica de examen de TAC (tomografía axial computerizada)
(ehl dohk-'tohr kee-'eh-reh ah-'sehr 'oon-ah 'tehk-nee-kah deh ehk-'sah-mehn de teh-ah-'seh (toh-moh-grah-'fee-ah ahk-see-'ahl kohm-poo-tehr-ee-'sah-dah))

To check your brain
Para examinar su cerebro
('pah-rah ehk-sah-mee-'nahr soo seh-'reh-broh)

To check your stomach
Para examinar su estómago
('pah-rah ehk-sah-mee-'nahr soo ehs-'toh-mah-goh)

To check your lungs
Para examinar sus pulmones
('pah-rah ehk-sah-mee-'nahr soos pool-'moh-nehs)

To check your liver
Para examinar su hígado
(p'ah-rah ehk-sah-mee-'nahr soo 'ee-gah-doh)

To check your sinuses
Para examinar sus senos nasales
('pah-rah ehk-sah-mee-'nahr soos 'see-nohs nah-'sahl-ehs)

You will need to drink this liquid at night
Va a necesitar tomarse este liquido en la noche
(bah ah neh-seh-see-'tahr toh-'mahr-seh 'ehs-teh lee-kee-doh ehn lah 'noh-cheh)

Before the test
Antes del examen
('ahn-tehs dehl ehk-'sah-mehn)

It is a laxative.
Es un laxativo.
(ehs oon lahk-sah-'tee-boh)

You need to drink these two glasses of contrast an hour before the test.
Va a necesitar tomarse estos dos vasos de contraste una hora antes del examen.
(bah ah neh-seh-see-'tahr toh-'mahr-seh 'ehs-tohs dohs 'bah-sohs deh kohn-'trah-steh 'oo-nah 'oh-rah 'ahn-tehs dehl ehk-'sah-mehn)

Take off your clothes.
Quítese la ropa.
('kee-teh-seh lah 'roh-pah)

Put this gown on.
Póngase esta bata.
('pohn-gah-seh 'ehs-tah 'bah-tah)

Take a deep breath.
Respire profundamente.
(rehs-'pee-reh proh-'foon-dah-'mehn-teh)

5

Hold it.
Deténgalo.
(deh-'tehn-gah-loh)

You can breathe now.
Puede respirar.
('pweh-deh rehs-pee-'rahr)

You are going to hear a strong noise.
Va a oir un ruido fuerte.
(bah ah oh-'eer oon roo-'ee-doh 'fwehr-teh)

Do not move.
No se mueva.
(noh seh 'mweh-bah)

I am going to inject this contrast.
Le voy a inyectar un contraste.
(leh boy ah een-yehk-'tahr oon kohn-'trahs-teh)

You may feel warm all over.
Puede darle calor.
('pweh-deh 'dahr-leh kah-'lohr)

But it is normal.
Pero es normal.
('peh-roh ehs nohr-'mahl)

Let me know
Déjeme saber
('deh-heh-meh sah-'behr)

If you cannot breathe
Si no puede respirar
(see noh 'pweh-deh rehs-pee-'rahr)

Or if you feel uncomfortable
O si se siente incómodo
(oh see seh see-'ehn-teh een-'koh-moh-doh)

Common Imaging Tests

I am going to take some X-rays of your
Voy a tomar unos rayos X de su
(boy ah toh-'mahr 'oo-nohs 'rah-yohs 'eh-kees deh soo)

Chest
Pecho
('peh-choh)

Abdomen
Abdomen
(ahb-'doh-mehn)

Head
Cabeza
(kah-'beh-sah)

Sinus
Senos nasales
('seh-nohs nah-'sah-lehs)

Extremities
Extremidades
(ehks-treh-mee-'dah-dehs)

Hand
Mano
('mah-noh)

Foot
Pie
(pee-'eh)

Fingers
Dedos
('deh-dohs)

KUB (Kidney / urethra / bladder)
Riñon-uretra-vejiga
(ree-'nyohn, oo-'reh-trah, beh-'hee-gah)

Your nurse practitioner / doctor has ordered a
Su enfermera / doctor ha ordenado un
(soo ehn-fehr-'meh-rah / dohk-'tohr ah ohr-deh-'nah-doh oon)

Computed Tomography (CT)
una técnica de examen TAC (Tomografia computorizada)
('oon-ah 'tehk-nee-kah deh ehk-'sah-mehn de teh-ah-'seh (toh-moh-grah-'fee-ah))

Magnetic Resonance Imaging (MRI)
Imagen de Resonancia Magnética (IRM)
(ee-'mah-hen deh reh-soh-'nahn-see-ah mag-'neh-tee-kah)

Ultrasound
Ultrasonido
(oohl-trah-soh-'nee-doh)

To better examine your
Para examinar mejor su
('pah-rah ehk-sah-mee-'nahr meh-'hohr soo)

Chest
Pecho
('peh-choh)

Abdomen
Abdomen
(ahb-'doh-mehn)

Head
Cabeza
(kah-'beh-sah)

Sinus
Senos nasales
('see-nohs nah-'sah-lehs)

5

Nursing Interventions 6

Offering comfort is perhaps one of the most characteristic features of nursing. Offering comfort in another language is characteristic of a sensitive nurse who is concerned with providing the best care possible. When offering comfort, gestures and a kind word can make a world of difference. This may be manifested by a simple explanation such as, ***Tómese esta medicina; es para su dolor*** (*'toh-meh-seh 'ehs-tah meh-dee-'see-nah, ehs 'pah-rah soo doh-'lohr*) (*Take this medicine, it is for your pain*).

➤ COMFORT MEASURES

Nursing Instructions

Take this medicine.
Tómese esta medicina.
(*'toh-meh-seh 'ehs-tah meh-dee-'see-nah*)

It is for your pain.
Es para su dolor.
(*ehs 'pah-rah soo doh-'lohr*)

It is for your stomach.
Es para su estómago.
(ehs 'pah-rah soo ehs-'toh-mah-goh)

It is for your heart.
Es para su corazón.
(ehs 'pah-rah soo koh-rah-'sohn)

It is for your headache.
Es para su dolor de cabeza.
(ehs 'pah-rah soo doh-'lohr deh kah-'beh-sah)

You will need to start walking today.
Necesita empezar a caminar hoy.
(neh-seh-'see-tah ehm-peh-'sahr ah kah-mee-'nahr 'oh-ee)

Tell me when you are ready.
Dígame cuando esté listo(a).
('dee-gah-meh 'kwahn-doh ehs-'teh 'lees-toh / 'lees-tah)

The physical therapist will help you.
El fisioterapista le va a ayudar.
(ehl fee-see-oh-teh-rah-'pees-tah leh bah ah ah-yoo-'dahr)

I will help you.
Yo le voy a ayudar.
(yoh leh boy ah ah-yoo-'dahr)

I will be back in an hour.
Volveré en una hora.
(bohl-beh-'reh ehn 'oo-nah 'oh-rah)

I will be back in a few minutes.
Volveré en unos minutos.
(bohl-beh-'reh ehn 'oo-nohs mee-'noo-tohs)

Are you ready to take a shower?
¿Está listo(a) para bañarse?
(eh-'stah 'lees-toh / 'lees-tah 'pah-rah bahn-'yahr-seh)

Here are your towels.
Aquí estan las toallas.
(ah-'kee ehs-'tahn lahs toh-'ah-yahs)

Do you prefer a bed bath?
¿Prefiere un baño de cama?
(preh-fee-'eh-reh oon 'bah-nyoh deh 'kah-mah)

You may brush your teeth.
Puede cepillarse los dientes.
('pweh-deh seh-pee-'yahr-seh lohs dee-'ehn-tehs)

Do not drink any water.
No tome agua.
(noh 'toh-meh 'ah-gwah)

Do not go the bathroom by yourself.
No puede ir al baño solo(a).
(noh 'pweh-deh eer ahl 'bah-nyoh 'soh-loh / 'soh-lah)

Here is the call light.
Aquí está el botón de llamada.
(ah-'kee ehs-'tah ehl boh-'tohn deh yah-'mah-dah)

Call me when you are ready to get up.
Llámeme cuando esté listo(a) para levantarse.
('yah-meh-meh 'kwahn-doh ehs-'teh 'lees-toh / 'lees-tah 'pah-rah leh-bahn-'tahr-seh)

Let me raise the bed.
Déjeme levantarlo(a) en la cama.
('deh-heh-meh leh-bahn-'tahr-loh / leh-bahn-'tahr-lah ehn lah 'kah-mah)

6

Bend your knees.
Doble sus rodillas.
('doh-bleh soos roh-'dee-yahs)

Push with your feet.
Empuje con sus pies.
(ehm-'poo-heh kohn soos pee-'ehs)

Do you need an extra blanket (pillow)?
¿Necesita otra cobija (almohada)?
(neh-seh-'see-tah 'oh-trah koh-'bee-hah) (ahl-moh-'ah-dah)

Common Patient Requests

I am cold.
Tengo frío.
('tehn-goh 'free-oh)

I am hot.
Tengo calor.
('tehn-goh kah-'lohr)

I have pain.
Tengo dolor.
('tehn-goh doh-'lohr)

In my stomach.
En mi estómago.
(ehn mee ehs-'toh-mah-goh)

In my hand.
En mi mano.
(ehn mee 'mah-noh)

In my foot.
En mi pie.
(ehn mee pee-'eh)

In my leg.
En mi pierna.
(ehn mee pee-'ehr-nah)

Where they did the operation.
Donde me hicieron la operación.
('dohn-deh meh ee-see-'eh-rohn lah oh-peh-rah-see-'ohn)

I have chest pain.
Tengo dolor en el pecho.
('tehn-goh doh-'lohr ehn ehl 'peh-choh)

I can't breathe.
No puedo respirar.
(noh 'pweh-doh rehs-pee-'rahr)

I need to go to the bathroom.
Necesito ir al baño.
(neh-seh-'see-toh eer ahl 'bahn-yoh)

I need the bedpan.
Necesito el bacín / chata.
(neh-seh-'see-toh ehl bah-'seen 'cha-tah)

I am hungry.
Tengo hambre.
('tehn-goh 'ahm-breh)

I am thirsty.
Tengo sed.
('tehn-goh sehd)

6

Do you have an extra blanket?
¿Tiene otra cobija / cobertor?
(tee-'eh-neh 'oh-trah koh-'bee-ha / koh-behr-'tohr)

Do you have an extra pillow?
¿Tiene otra almohada?
(tee-'eh-neh 'oh-trah ahl-moh-'ah-dah)

Can I brush my teeth?
¿Puedo cepillarme los dientes?
('pweh-doh seh-pee-'yahr-meh lohs dee-'ehn-tehs)

I need my _____.
Necesito mi / mis _____.
(neh-seh-'see-toh mee / mees)

Walker.
Andadera.
(ahn-dah-'deh-rah)

Cane.
Bastón.
(bahs-'tohn)

Crutches.
Muletas.
(moo-'leh-tahs)

➤ *MEDICATION INSTRUCTIONS*

Oral Medications

Take one of these pills.
Tómese una de estas pastillas.
('toh-meh-seh 'oo-nah deh 'ehs-tahs pahs-'tee-yahs)

Once a day.
Una vez al día.
('oo-nah behs ahl 'dee-ah)

Twice a day.
Dos veces al día.
(dohs 'beh-sehs ahl 'dee-ah)

Three times a day.
Tres veces al día.
(trehs 'beh-sehs ahl 'dee-ah)

With food.
Con comida.
(kohn koh-'mee-dah)

Without food.
Sin comida.
(seen koh-'mee-dah)

Cut in half.
Córtela por la mitad.
('kohr-teh-lah pohr lah mee-'tahd)

Take one spoonful.
Tómese una cucharada.
('toh-meh-seh 'oo-nah koo-chah-'rah-dah)

Take half a spoonful.
Tómese media cucharada
('toh-meh-seh 'meh-dee-ah koo-chah-'rah-dah)

Take one capsule.
Tómese una cápsula.
('toh-meh-seh 'oo-nah 'kahp-soo-lah)

Put it under your tongue.
Póngala debajo de la lengua.
('pohn-gah-lah deh-'bah-hoh deh lah 'lehn-gwah)

And let it melt.
Y deje que se derrita.
(ee 'deh-heh keh seh deh-'ree-tah)

Injectables

You will need to inject your insulin ____.
Necesita inyectarse insulina ____.
(neh-seh-'see-tah een-yehk-'tahr-seh een-soo-'lee-nah)

Twice a day
Dos veces al día
(dohs 'beh-sehs ahl 'dee-ah)

Before meals
Antes de las comidas
('ahn-tehs deh lahs koh-'mee-dahs)

After checking your blood sugar
Después de verificar su nível de azúcar
(dehs-'pwehs deh vehr-ee-fee-'kahr soo nee-'behl deh ah-'soo-kahr)

As instructed by the doctor
Como se lo indicó el doctor
('koh-moh seh loh een-dee-'koh ehl dohk-'tohr)

Number of units of regular insulin
Número de unidades de insulina regular
('noo-meh-roh deh oo-nee-'dah-dehs deh een-soo-'lee-nah reh-goo-'lahr)

Number of units of NPH insulin
Número de unidades de insulina NPH
('noo-meh-roh deh oo-nee-'dah-dehs deh een-soo-'lee-nah 'eh-neh peh 'ah-cheh)

Draw the clear insulin first.
Saque primero la insulina clara.
('sah-keh pree-'meh-roh lah een-soh-'lee-nah 'klah-rah)

And then the cloudy one
Y luego la turbia
(ee 'lweh-goh lah 'toor-bee-ah)

Rotate the sites of the injection to your
Cambie los sitios de inyección al
('kahm-bee-eh lohs 'see-tee-ohs deh een-yehk-see-'ohn ahl)

Arm
Brazo
('brah-soh)

Abdomen
Estómago (abdomen)
(ehs-'toh-mah-goh) (ahb-'doh-mehn)

Thighs
Muslos
('moos-lohs)

Intravenous (IV)

I am going to start an IV
Voy a empezarle una venoclisis /venipuntura / intravenosa
(boy ah ehm-peh-'sahr-leh 'oo-nah beh-noh-'clee-sees / beh-nee-

poon-'too-rah / een-trah-beh-'noh-sah)

On your arm.
En su brazo
(ehn soo 'brah-soh)

It may hurt a little.
Puede doler un poco
('pweh-deh doh-'lehr oon 'poh-koh)

I am going to give you your medication
Le voy a dar su medicamento
(leh boy ah dahr soo meh-dee-kah-'mehn-toh)

Through your IV
En su venoclisis
(ehn soo beh-noh-'clee-sees)

Every 8 hours
Cada ocho horas
('kah-dah 'oh-choh 'oh-rahs)

It is an antibiotic.
Es un antibiótico.
(ehs oon ahn-tee-bee-'oh-tee-koh)

It is chemotherapy.
Es quimioterapia.
(ehs kee-mee-oh-teh-'rah-pee-ah)

Call me if you feel uncomfortable.
Llámeme si se siente incómodo.
('yah-meh-meh see seh see-'ehn-teh een-'koh-moh-doh)

Call me if you feel any pain
Llámeme si siente algún dolor
('yah-meh-meh see see-'ehn-teh ahl-'goon doh-'lohr)

6

At the IV site
En el sitio de la venoclisis
(ehn ehl 'see-tee-oh deh lah beh-noh-'clee-sees)

If you are short of breath
Si le falta la respiración
(see leh 'fahl-tah lah rehs-pee-rah-see-'ohn)

Or if you have chest pains
O si tiene dolor de pecho
(oh see tee-'eh-neh doh-'lohr deh 'peh-choh)

➤ *DISCHARGE INSTRUCTIONS*

Call your doctor for an appointment
Llame a su médico para una cita
('yah-meh ah soo 'meh-dee-koh 'pah-rah 'oo-nah 'see-tah)

Next week
La semana que viene
(lah seh-'mah-nah keh bee-'ehn-eh)

In three days
En tres días
(ehn trehs 'dee-ahs)

In a month
En un mes
(ehn oon mehs)

This is your doctor's phone number.
Éste es el número de télefono de su médico.
('ehs-teh ehs ehl 'noo-meh-roh deh teh-'leh-foh-noh deh soo 'meh-dee-koh)

6

Eat only liquids.
Tome solamente líquidos.
('toh-meh soh-lah-'mehn-teh 'lee-kee-dohs)

Use your cane.
Use su bastón.
('oo-seh soo bahs-'tohn)

Walker
Andadera
(ahn-dah-'deh-rah)

Crutches
Muletas
(moo-'leh-tahs)

Oxygen
Oxígeno
(ohk-'see-heh-noh)

Call your doctor if you notice
Llame a su médico si nota
('yah-meh ah soo 'meh-dee-koh see 'noh-tah)

Fever
Fiebre
(fee-'eh-breh)

Pain
Dolor
(doh-'lohr)

Swelling
Hinchazón
(een-chah-'sohn)

Redness
Enrojecimiento
(ehn-roh-heh-see-mee-'ehn-toh)

Discharge
Desecho
(dehs-'eh-choh)

On the wound
En la herida
(ehn lah eh-'ree-dah)

In the Emergency Room

7

Emergencies are a stressful time for any person, let alone for someone who is not able to communicate appropriately without assistance. In the emergency room, nurses must tend to the most immediate need of the patient, while attempting to provide care that is sensitive and culturally appropriate. Practice the questions most frequently used in your setting so you become thoroughly familiar with the pronunciation. This exercise will come in handy when there is not enough time to look in a book to find the most appropriate way of communicating with a client.

➤ FRONT DESK / TRIAGE

How can I help you?
¿Cómo le puedo ayudar?
(ʻkoh-moh leh ʻpweh-doh ah-yoo-ʻdahr)

Cardiac

I have chest pain.
Tengo dolor de pecho.
(ʻtehn-goh doh-ʻlohr deh ʻpeh-choh)

I feel chest pressure.
Siento presión en el pecho.
(see-'ehn-toh preh-see-'ohn ehn-ehl 'peh-choh)

I am short of breath.
Estoy sofocado.
(eh-'stoy soh-foh-'kah-doh)

When did it start?
¿Cuándo empezó?
('kwahn-doh ehm-peh-'soh)

When did it get worse?
¿Cuándo empeoró?
('kwahn-doh ehm-peh-ohr-'oh)

Do you have angina?
¿Tiene angina?
(tee-'eh-neh ahn-'hee-nah)

Abdominal

I have stomach pain.
Tengo dolor del estómago.
('tehn-goh doh-'lohr dehl ehs-'toh-mah-goh)

Do you have any blood in your stool?
¿Tiene sangre en el excremento?
(tee-'eh-neh 'sahn-greh ehn ehl ehks-kreh-'mehn-toh)

Are you nauseated?
¿Tiene náusea?
(tee-'eh-neh 'nahw-seh-ah)

Have you been vomiting?
¿Ha estado vomitando?
(ah ehs-'tah-doh boh-mee-'tahn-doh)

Neurological

I feel weak.
Me siento débil.
(meh see-'ehn-toh 'deh-beel)

I feel faint.
Siento que me voy a desmayar.
(see-'ehn-toh keh meh boy ah dehs-mah-'yahr)

She / he fainted.
Ella / él se desmayó.
('eh-yah / ehl seh dehs-mah-'yoh)

I have blurred vision.
Tengo la visión borrosa.
('tehn-goh lah bee-see-'ohn boh-'rroh-sah)

I have a headache.
Tengo dolor de cabeza.
('tehn-goh doh-'lohr deh kah-'beh-sah)

She / he is not able to speak.
Ella / él no puede hablar.
('eh-yah / ehl noh 'pweh-deh ah-'blahr)

➤ ACCIDENTS

What happened?
¿Qué pasó?
(keh pah-'soh)

At what time?
¿A qué hora?
(ah keh 'oh-rah)

7

Did you pass out?
¿Se desmayó?
(she dehs-mah-'yoh)

Were you driving?
¿Estaba usted manejando?
(ehs-'tah-bah oo-'stehd mah-neh-'hahn-doh)

How fast were you going?
¿Qué rápido fue?
(keh 'rah-pee-doh fweh)

Were you wearing a seatbelt?
¿Llevaba puesto el cinturón de seguridad?
(yeh-'bah-bah 'pwehs-toh ehl seen-too-'rohn deh seh-goo-ree-'dahd)

Did you get out of the car by yourself?
¿Usted pudo salir del carro sin ayuda?
(oo'stehd 'poo-doh sah-'leer dehl 'kah-rroh seen ah-'yoo-dah)

➤ STABBING / GUNSHOT WOUNDS

When did you get stabbed / shot?
¿Cuándo le acuchillaron /dispararon?
('kwahn-doh leh ah-koo-chee-'yah-rohn / dees-pah-'rah-rohn)

How many times?
¿Cuántas veces?
('kwahn-tahs 'beh-sehs)

What kind of knife / gun?
¿Qué tipo de cuchillo / arma?
(keh 'tee-poh deh koo-'chee-yoh / 'ahr-mah)

Were there any other people involved?
¿Hubo otra gente afectada?
(*'oo-boh 'oh-trah 'hen-teh ah-fehk-'tah-dah*)

Do you have a relative we can contact?
¿Tiene algún familiar que podamos llamar?
(*tee-'eh-neh ahl-'goon fah-mee-lee-'ahr keh poh-'dah-mohs yah-'mahr*)

Who can we call?
¿A quién podemos llamar?
(*ah kee-'ehn poh-'deh-mos yah-'mahr*)

What's the phone number?
¿Cuál es su número de teléfono?
(*kwahl ehs soo 'noo-meh-roh deh teh-'leh-foh-noh*)

What's the address?
¿Cuál es su dirección?
(*kwahl ehs soo dee-rehk-see-'ohn*)

Are you allergic to any medications?
¿Es usted alérgico a algún medicamento?
(*ehs oo-'stehd ah-'lehr-hee-koh ah ahl-'goon meh-dee-kah-'mehn-toh*)

We are going to start an IV.
Vamos a empezar una venoclisis.
(*'bah-mohs ah ehm-peh-'sahr 'oo-nah beh-noh-'clee-sees*)

We are going to put you on oxygen.
Le vamos a poner oxígeno.
(*leh 'bah-mohs ah poh-'nehr ohk-'see-heh-noh*)

7

We are going to take you to the operating room.
Le vamos a llevar a la sala de operaciones.
(leh 'bah-mohs ah yeh-'bahr ah lah 'sah-lah deh oh-peh-rah-see-'oh-nehs)

We are going to sedate you.
Le vamos a administrar una sedativa.
(leh 'bah-mohs ah ahd-mee-nee-'strahr 'oo-nah seh-dah-'tee-vah)

We are going to put a tube down your throat to help you breathe.
Le vamos a poner un tubo en la garganta para ayudarle a respirar.
(leh 'bah-mohs ah poh-'nehr oon 'too-boh ehn lah gahr-'gahn-tah 'pah-rah ah-yoo-'dahr-leh ah rehs-pee-'rahr)

Have you ever had any major surgeries?
¿Le han hecho alguna cirugía?
(leh ahn 'eh-choh ahl-'goo-nah see-roo-'hee-ah)

We are going to take X-rays.
Le vamos a llevar al departamento de rayos X.
(leh 'bah-mohs ah yeh-'bahr ahl deh-pahr-tah-'mehn-toh de 'rah-yohs 'eh-kees)

We are going to do a CT (computed tomagraphy) scan
Vamos a tomar un TAC (tomografía axial computerizada)
('bah-mohs ah toh-'mahr oon teh ah seh)

To check for any internal damages
Para ver si hay heridas internas
('pah-rah behr see 'ah-ee ehr-'ee-dahs een-'tehr-nahs)

To your stomach
A su estómago
(ah soo ehs-'toh-mah-goh)

To your lungs
A sus pulmones
(ah soos pool-'moh-nehs)

To your brain
A su cerebro
(ah soo seh-'reh-broh)

We are here to help you.
Estamos aquí para ayudarle.
(eh-'stah-mohs ah-'kee 'pah-rah ah-yoo-'dahr-leh)

Do not be scared.
No tenga miedo.
(noh 'tehn-gah mee-'eh-doh)

➤ POISONING

What did you take?
¿Qué tomó?
(keh toh-'moh)

What did your son / daughter take?
¿Qué tomó su hijo / hija?
(keh toh-'moh soo 'ee-hoh / 'ee-hah)

Do you have the bottle?
¿Tiene la botella?
(tee-'eh-neh lah boh-'teh-yah)

How much did you / he / she take?
¿Cuánto tomó?
('kwahn-toh toh-'moh)

Half a bottle?
¿Media botella?
('meh-dee-ah boh-'teh-yah)

A whole bottle?
¿La botella entera?
(lah boh-'teh-yah ehn-'teh-rah)

How many pills?
¿Cuántas pastillas?
('kwahn-tahs pahs-'tee-yahs)

How long ago?
¿Hace cuánto tiempo?
('ah-seh 'kwahn-toh tee-'ehm-poh)

Do you have any trouble breathing?
¿Tiene algunos problemas para respirar?
(tee-'eh-neh ahl-'goon-ohs proh-'bleh-mahs 'pah-rah rehs-pee-'rahr)

Do you have any pain?
¿Tiene dolor?
(tee-'eh-neh doh-'lohr)

Did you vomit?
¿Ha vomitado?
(ah boh-mee-'tah-doh)

Are you nauseated?
¿Tiene nausea?
(tee-'eh-neh 'nahw-seh-ah)

Do you have a headache?
¿Tiene dolor de cabeza?
(tee-'ehn-eh doh-'lohr de kah-'beh-sah)

7

Do you have a stomachache?
¿Tiene dolor de estómago?
(tee-'ehn-eh doh-'lohr deh ehs-'toh-mah-goh)

Did you call the poison control center?
¿Llamó al centro de envenenamiento?
(yah-'moh ahl 'sehn-troh deh ehn-beh-neh-nah-mee-'ehn-toh)

What did they say?
¿Qué le dijeron?
(keh leh dee-'heh-rohn)

➤ *WOUNDS*

When was your last tetanus shot?
¿Cuándo fué su última vacuna para el tétano?
('kwahn-doh fweh soo 'ool-tee-mah bah-'koo-nah 'pah-rah ehl 'teh-tah-noh)

How did you cut yourself?
¿Cómo se cortó?
('koh-moh seh kohr-'toh)

Cutting vegetables
Cortando vegetales
(kohr-'tahn-doh beh-heh-'tah-lehs)

Playing with a knife
Jugando con un cuchillo
(hoo-'gahn-doh kohn oon koo-'chee-yoh)

I stepped on a nail
He pisado un clavo
(eh pee-'sah-doh oon 'klah-boh)

7

Arguing with my husband
Discutiendo con mi esposo
(dees-koo-tee-'ehn-doh kohn mee ehs-'poh-soh)

Wife
Esposa
(ehs-'poh-sah)

Partner
Pareja
(pah-'reh-ha)

Girlfriend
Novia
('noh-bee-ah)

Boyfriend
Novio
('noh-bee-oh)

➤ *SEXUAL ASSAULT / DOMESTIC VIOLENCE*

How did the assault / attack take place?
¿Cómo occurrió el asalto / ataque?
('koh-moh oh-koo-ree-'oh ehl ah-'sahl-toh / ah-'tah-keh)

Where did the assault / attack take place?
¿Dónde occurrió el asalto / ataque?
('dohn-deh oh-koo-ree-'oh ehl ah-'sahl-toh / ah-'tah-keh)

At home
En la casa / En el hogar
(ehn lah 'kah-sah / ehn ehl oh-'gahr)

At a bar
En un bar
(ehn oon bahr)

On the street
En la calle
(ehn lah 'kah-yeh)

At work
En el trabajo
(ehn ehl trah-'bah-hoh)

Did more than one person assault you?
¿Fue más de una persona que le atacó?
(fweh mahs deh 'oo-nah pehr-'soh-nah keh leh ah-tah-'koh)

How many?
¿Cuántos / Cuántas?
('kwahn-tohs / 'kwahn-tahs)

Have you been assaulted / attacked by
Le han asaltado / atacado antes por
(leh ahn ah-sahl-'tah-doh / ah-tah-'kah-doh 'ahn-tehs pohr)

This person before?
¿Esa persona?
('eh-sah pehr-'soh-nah)

These people before?
¿Esas personas?
('eh-sahs pehr-'soh-nahs)

What is your relationship with this person?
¿Cuál es su relación con esta persona?
(kwahl ehs soo reh-lah-see-'ohn kohn 'ehs-tah pehr-'soh-nah)

7

Is he your husband?
¿Es su esposo?
(ehs soo ehs-'poh-soh)

Is she your wife?
¿Es su esposa?
(ehs soo ehs-'poh-sah)

Partner?
¿Pareja?
(pah-'reh-hah)

Friend?
¿Amigo?
(ah-'mee-goh)

Co-worker?
¿Compañero de trabajo?
(kohm-pahn-'yehr-oh deh trah-'bah-hoh)

Family member?
¿Familiar?
(fah-mee-lee-'ahr)

Customer?
¿Cliente?
(klee-'ehn-teh)

Stranger?
¿Alguien que no conoce?
('ahl-gee-ehn keh noh koh-'noh-seh)

What were you attacked with?
¿Con qué fue atacado?
(kohn keh fweh ah-tah-'kah-doh)

With a knife?
¿Con un cuchillo?
(kohn oon koo-'chee-yoh)

With a firearm?
¿Con una arma de fuego?
(kohn oonah 'ahr-mah deh 'fweh-goh)

With a piece of glass?
¿Con un pedazo de vidrio?
(kohn un peh-'dah-soh deh 'bee-dree-oh)

With a bottle?
¿Con una botella?
(kohn oonah boh-'teh-yah)

Why did she / he attack you?
¿Porqué le atacó a usted?
(pohr-'keh leh ah-tah-'koh ah oo-'stehd)

Sexual reasons?
¿Razones sexuales?
(rah-'soh-nehs sehk-soo-'ah-lehs)

Racial reasons?
¿Razones raciales?
(rah-'soh-nehs rah-see-'ah-lehs)

Theft?
¿Robo?
('roh-boh)

Personal argument?
¿Discusión personal?
(dees-koo-see-'ohn pehr-soh-'nahl)

Did you report this assault to the police?
¿Reportó usted el asalto a la policia?
(reh-'pohr-toh oo-stehd ehl ah-'sahl-toh ah lah poh-'lee-see-ah)

Please, tell me about your
Por favor, dígame acerca de su
(pohr fah-'bohr 'dee-gah-meh ah-'sehr-kah deh soo)

Headache
Dolor de cabeza
(doh-'lohr deh kah-'beh-sah)

Chest pain
Dolor del pecho
(doh-'lohr dehl 'peh-choh)

Fever
Fiebre
(fee-'eh-breh)

Abdominal pain
Dolor abdominal / Dolor del estómago
(doh-'lohr ahb-doh-mee-'nahl / doh-'lohr dehl ehs-'toh-mah-goh)

Blurred vision
Visión borrosa
(bee-see-'ohn boh-'rroh-sah)

Dizziness
Mareo
(mah-'reh-oh)

Leg pain
Dolor de pierna
(doh-'lohr deh pee-'ehr-nah)

Shortness of breath
Sofocamiento / falta de respiración
(soh-foh-kah-mee-'ehn-toh / 'fahl-tah deh rehs-pee-rah-see-'ohn)

➤ *PAIN ASSESSMENT*

P: *Provocative*

What causes the pain?
¿Qué le causa el dolor?
(keh leh 'kahw-sah ehl doh-'lohr)

Food
La comida / los alimentos
(lah koh-'mee-dah / lohs ah-lee-'mehn-tohs)

Breathing deeply
Respiraciones profundas
(rehs-pee-rah-see-'oh-nehs pro-'foon-dahs)

Exercise
El ejercicio
(ehl eh-hehr-'see-see-oh)

What makes the pain worse?
¿Qué empeora el dolor?
(keh leh ehm-peh-ohr-ah ehl doh-'lohr)

Food
La comida / los alimentos
(lah koh-'mee-dah / lohs ahl-ee-'mehn-tohs)

Deep breaths
Respiraciones profundas
(rehs-pee-rah-see-'oh-nehs pro-'foon-dahs)

Exercise
El ejercicio
(ehl eh-hehr-'see-see-oh)

Standing
Estar de pie
(eh-'stahr deh pee-'eh)

Bending
Doblarse
(doh-'blahr-seh)

Lying down
Acostarse
(ah-cos-'tahr-seh)

Walking
Caminar
(kah-mee-'nahr)

Running
Correr
(koh-'rrehr)

What makes the pain better?
¿Qué le mejora el dolor?
(keh leh meh-'hohr-ah ehl doh-'lohr)

Medication
Medicamento
(meh-dee-kah-'mehn-toh)

Rest
Descanso
(dehs-'kahn-soh)

Cold
El frío
(ehl 'free-oh)

Warmth
El calor
(ehl kah-'lohr)

Food
La comida / los alimentos
(lah koh-'mee-dah / lohs ah-lee-'mehn-tohs)

Deep breaths
Respiraciones profundas
(rehs-pee-rah-see-'oh-nehs pro-'foon-dahs)

Exercising
El ejercicio
(ehl eh-hehr-'see-see-oh)

Standing
Estar de pie
(eh-'stahr deh pee-'eh)

Bending
Doblarse
(doh-'blahr-seh)

Lying down
Acostarse
(ah-cost-'ahr-seh)

7

Walking
Caminar
(kah-mee-'nahr)

Running
Correr
(koh-'rrehr)

Q: *Quality or Quantity*

Do you have pain?
¿Tiene dolor?
(tee-'eh-neh doh-'lohr)

How does it feel?
¿Cómo lo siente?
('koh-moh loh see-'ehn-teh)

Describe your pain:
Describa su dolor:
(dehs-'kre-bah soo doh-'lohr)

Acute?
¿Agudo?
(ah-'goo-doh)

Burning?
¿Le quema?
(leh 'keh-mah)

Comes and goes?
¿Va y viene?
(bah ee bee-'eh-neh)

Does it bother you?
¿Le molesta?
(leh moh-'lehs-tah)

R: *Region or Radiation*

Where do you have your pain?
¿Dónde tiene el dolor?
('dohn-deh tee-'eh-neh ehl doh-'lohr)

In my head
En la cabeza
(ehn lah kah-'beh-sah)

In my ears
En los oidos
(ehn lohs oh-'ee-dohs)

In my eyes
En los ojos
(ehn lohs 'oh-hohs)

In my mouth
En la boca
(ehn lah 'boh-kah)

In my tooth (teeth)
En el diente / en los dientes
(ehn ehl dee-'ehn-teh / ehn lohs dee-'ehn-tehs)

In my throat
En la garganta
(ehn lah gahr-'gahn-tah)

In my chest
En el pecho
(ehn ehl 'peh-choh)

In my arms
En los brazos
(ehn lohs 'brah-sohs)

In my hands
En las manos
(ehn lahs 'mah-nohs)

In my fingers
En los dedos
(ehn lohs 'deh-dohs)

In my fingernail / fingernails
En la uña / en las uñas
(ehn lah 'oon-yah / ehn lahs 'oon-yahs)

In my stomach
En el estómago
(ehn ehl ehs-'toh-mah-goh)

In my womb
En la matriz
(ehn lah mah-'trees)

In my penis
En el pene
(ehn ehl 'peh-neh)

In my legs
En las piernas
(ehn lahs pee-'ehr-nahs)

In my feet
En los pies
(ehn lohs pee-'ehs)

In my toes
En los dedos de los pies
(ehn lohs 'deh-dohs deh lohs pee-'ehs)

Where does it go?
¿A dónde se va?
(ah 'dohn-deh seh bah)

To the left arm
Al brazo izquierdo
(ahl 'brah-soh ees-kee-'ehr-doh)

To the throat
Al cuello
(ahl 'kweh-yoh)

To my right side
A mi lado derecho
(ah mee 'lah-doh deh-'reh-choh)

To my left side
A mi lado izquierdo
(ah mee 'lah-doh ees-kee-'ehr-doh)

Below
Para abajo
('pah-rah ah-'bah-hoh)

Above
Para arriba
('pah-rah ah-'rree-bah)

7

S: *Severity Scale*

If zero means no pain, and ten means the greatest pain you have ever had, what number do you give your pain?
Si cero es ningún dolor, y diez el dolor más fuerte que haya tenido, ¿qué número le da a su dolor?
(see 'seh-roh ehs neen-'goon doh-'lohr, ee 'dee-ehs ehl doh-'lohr mahs 'fwehr-teh keh 'hah-yah teh-'nee-doh, keh 'noo-meh-roh leh dah ah soo doh-'lohr)

How much pain do you have?
¿Cuánto dolor tiene?
('Kwahn-toh doh-'lohr tee-'eh-neh)

Little (very little)
Poco (poquito)
('po-koh) (poh-'kee-toh)

A moderate amount
Moderado (más o menos)
(moh-deh-'rah-doh) (mahs oh 'meh-nohs)

A lot
Mucho
('moo-choh)

T: *Timing*

When did it first happen?
¿Cuándo le pasó por primera vez?
('kwahn-doh leh pah-'soh pohr pree-'meh-rah behs)

Yesterday
Ayer
(ah-'yehr)

Seven hours ago
Hace siete horas
('ah-seh see-'eh-teh 'oh-rahs)

Two days ago
Hace dos días
('ah-seh dohs 'dee-ahs)

Three weeks ago
Hace tres semanas
('ah-seh trehs seh-'mah-nahs)

Four months ago
Hace cuatro meses
('ah-seh 'kwa-troh 'meh-sehs)

A year ago
Hace un año
('ah-seh oon 'ahn-yoh)

In the morning
En la mañana
(ehn lah mah-'nyah-nah)

Yesterday evening
Ayer por la tarde
(ah-'yehr pohr lah 'tahr-deh)

Last night
Anoche
(ah-'noh-cheh)

How long does it last?
¿Por cuánto tiempo le dura?
(pohr 'kwahn-toh tee-'ehm-poh leh 'doo-rah)

7

About fifteen minutes
Como quince minutos
('koh-moh 'keen-seh mee-'noo-tohs)

About an hour
Como una hora
('koh-moh 'oo-nah 'oh-rah)

How often does it happen?
¿Con cuál frecuencia le pasa?
(kohn kwahl freh-'kwen-see-ah leh 'pah-sah)

Every time I eat
Cada vez que como
('kah-dah behs keh 'koh-moh)

Every time I go to the bathroom
Cada vez que voy al baño
('kah-dah behs keh boy ahl 'bah-nyoh)

Every time I get upset
Cada vez que me enojo
('kah-dah behs keh meh eh-'noh-hoh)

Every time I walk
Cada vez que camino
('kah-dah behs keh kah-'mee-noh)

Every time I bend down
Cada vez que me agacho
('kah-dah behs keh meh ah-'gah-choh)

Every time I stand up
Cada vez que me pongo de pie
('kah-dah behs keh meh 'pohn-goh deh pee-'eh)

When I lie down
Cuando me acuesto
('kwahn-doh meh ah-'kwehs-toh)

When I get up
Cuando me levanto
('kwahn-doh meh leh-'bahn-toh)

U: *Understand Patient's Perception*

What do you think it is?
¿Qué piensa usted que sea?
(keh pee-'ehn-sah oo-'stehd keh 'seh-ah)

Cancer
Cáncer
('kahn-sehr)

Diabetes
Diabetes
(de-ah-'beh-tehs)

High blood pressure
Alta presión
('ahl-tah preh-see-'ohn)

Gastritis
Gastritis
(gahs-'tree-tees)

Stroke
Embolia
(ehm-'boh-lee-ah)

7

Tumor
Tumor
(too-'mohr)

I do not know.
No sé.
(noh seh)

Fright
Susto
('soos-toh)

Rage
Coraje
(koh-'rah-heh)

Witchcraft
Embrujo
(ehm-'broo-hoh)

Evil eye
Mal de ojo
(mahl deh 'oh-hoh)

➤ *PAST MEDICAL HISTORY*

Have you had _____?
¿Ha tenido _____?
(ah teh-'nee-doh)

Measles
Sarampión
(sah-rahm-pee-'ohn)

Mumps
Paperas
(pah-'peh-rahs)

Rubella
Rubéola
(roo-'beh-oh-lah)

Chicken pox
Varicella
(bah-ree-'seh-lah)

Scarlet fever
Fiebre escarlatina
(fee-'eh-breh ehs-kahr-lah-'tee-nah)

Poliomyelitis
Poliomelitis
(poh-lee-oh-meh-'lee-tees)

Rheumatic fever
Fiebre reumática
(fee-'eh-breh reh-oo-'mah-tee-kah)

Automobile accident
Accidente de auto
(ahk-see-'dehn-teh deh 'ow-toh)

Fractures
Fracturas
(frahk-'too-rahs)

Wounds
Heridas
(eh-'ree-dahs)

Head contusions
Contusiones en la cabeza
(kohn-too-see-'oh-nehs ehn lah kah-'beh-sah)

Burns
Quemaduras
(keh-mah-'doo-rahs)

Diabetes
Diabetes
(de-ah-'beh-tehs)

Hypertension
Presión alta
(preh-see-'ohn 'ahl-tah)

Heart disease
Enfermedades del corazón
(ehn-fehr-meh-'dah-dehs dehl koh-rah-'sohn)

Cancer
Cáncer
('kahn-sehr)

7

Have you been hospitalized?
¿Ha estado alguna vez hospitalizado?
(ah ehs-'tah-doh ahl-'goo-nah behs ohs-pee-tahl-ee-'sah-doh)

Have you ever had surgery?
¿Ha tenido alguna cirugía?
(ah teh-'nee-doh ahl-'goo-nah see-roo-'hee-ah)

What kind?
¿Qué tipo?
(keh 'tee-poh)

Appendix
Apéndice
(ah-'pehn-dee-seh)

Stomach
Estómago
(ehs-'toh-mah-goh)

Heart
Corazón
(koh-rah-'sohn)

Spleen
Bazo
('bah-soh)

Hernia
Hernia
('ehr-nee-ah)

Hysterectomy
Histerectomía
(ees-teh-rehk-toh-'mee-ah)

Cesarean section
Sección cesárea
(sehk-see-'ohn ceh-'sah-ree-ah)

➤ *INSTRUCTIONS TO PATIENTS*

The doctor thinks you have
El doctor piensa que tiene
(ehl dohk-'tohr pee-'ehn-sah keh tee-'eh-neh)

Pneumonia
Neumonía
(neh-oo-moh-'nee-ah)

Gastritis
Gastritis
(gahs-'tree-tees)

Gallstones
Piedras en la vesícula
(pee-'eh-drahs ehn lah bee-'see-koo-lah)

Anxiety
Ansiedad
(ahn-see-eh-'dahd)

Asthma
Asma
('ahs-mah)

Bronchitis
Bronquitis
(brohn-'kee-tees)

Cancer
Cáncer
('kahn-sehr)

Diabetes
Diabetes
(dee-ah-'beh-tehs)

Hypertension
Presión alta
(preh-see-'ohn 'ahl-tah)

Angina
Angina de pecho
(ahn-'hee-nah deh 'peh-choh)

A broken bone
Un hueso fracturado
(oon 'weh-soh frahk-too-'rah-doh)

An ankle sprain
Una torcedura de tobillo
('oo-nah tohr-seh-'doo-rah deh toh-'bee-yoh)

A broken hip
Una cadera fracturada
('oo-nah kah-'deh-rah frahk-too-'rah-dah)

Stomach infection
Infección del estómago
(een-fehk-see-'ohn dehl ehs-'toh-mah-goh)

Infection in your throat
Infección en la garganta
(een-fehk-see-'ohn ehn lah gahr-'gahn-tah)

Make an appointment to see your doctor
Haga una cita con su doctor
('ah-gah 'oo-nah 'see-tah kohn soo dohk-'tohr)

In three days.
En tres días.
(ehn trehs 'dee-ahs)

In two weeks.
En dos semanas.
(ehn dohs seh-'mah-nahs)

7

Call 911

Llame al nueve uno uno

('yah-meh ahl noo-'eh-beh 'oo-noh 'oo-noh)

Return to the emergency department

Regrese al departamento de emergencias

(reh-'greh-seh ahl deh-pahr-tah-'mehn-toh deh eh-mehr-'hehn-see-ahs)

If you get worse.

Si se empeora.

(see seh ehm-peh-'oh-rah)

If you don't get better.

Si no se mejora.

(see noh seh meh-'hoh-rah)

If it happens again.

Si pasa de nuevo.

(see 'pah-sah deh noo-'eh-boh)

If you get a fever.

Si tiene fiebre.

(see tee-'eh-neh fee-'eh-breh)

To have your sutures / staples removed.

Para remover sus suturas / grapas.

('pah-rah reh-moh-'behr soos soo-'too-rahs / 'grah-pahs)

In 7 days.

En siete días.

(ehn see-'eh-teh 'dee-ahs)

To check on your infection.

Para examinar su infección.

('pah-rah ehk-sah-mee-'nahr soo een-fehk-see-'ohn)

In 3 days.
En tres días.
(ehn trehs 'dee-ahs)

Take this pill
Tome esta píldora
('toh-meh 'ehs-tah 'peel-doh-rah)

Twice a day.
Dos veces al día.
(dohs 'beh-sehs ahl 'dee-ah)

Three times a day.
Tres veces al día.
(trehs 'beh-sehs ahl 'dee-ah)

Until it is gone.
Hasta que se acabe.
('ah-stah keh seh ah-'kah-beh)

Until you see your doctor.
Hasta que vea a su médico.
('ah-stah keh 'beh-ah ah soo 'meh-dee-koh)

Keep the cast dry.
Mantenga el yeso seco.
(mahn-'tehn-gah ehl 'yes-oh 'seh-koh)

Use the crutches at all times.
Use las muletas todo el tiempo.
('oo-seh lahs moo-'leh-tahs 'toh-doh ehl tee-'ehm-poh)

Do not bear any weight on that leg.
No ponga ningún peso en esa pierna.
(noh 'pohn-gah neen-'goon 'peh-soh ehn 'eh-sah pee-'ehr-nah)

7

Keep the wound clean and dry.
Mantenga la herida limpia y seca.
(mahn-'tehn-gah lah eh-'ree-dah 'leem-pee-ah ee 'seh-kah)

Change the dressing once a day.
Cambie la venda una vez al día.
('kahm-bee-eh lah 'behn-dah 'oo-nah behs ahl 'dee-ah)

➤ *ITEMS / PEOPLE FOUND IN THE EMERGENCY ROOM*

Gurney
Camilla
(kah-'mee-yah)

Wheelchair
Silla de ruedas
('see-yah deh rweh-dahs)

Waiting room
Sala de espera
('sah-lah deh ehs-'peh-rah)

Patient room
Cuarto de paciente
('kwahr-toh deh pah-see-'ehn-teh)

Radiology department
Departamento de radiología
(deh-pahr-tah-'mehn-toh deh rah-dee-oh-loh-'hee-ah)

Nurses' station
Estación de enfermeras
(ehs-tah-see-'ohn deh ehn-fehr-'meh-rahs)

Cafeteria
Cafetería
(kah-feh-teh-'ree-ah)

Medical chart
Expediente
(ehks-peh-dee-'ehn-teh)

Medical records
Expedientes / registro de expedientes
(ehks-peh-dee-'ehn-tehs / reh-'hees-troh deh ehks-peh-dee-'ehn-tehs)

Observation room
Cuarto de observaciones
('kwahr-toh deh ohb-sehr-bah-see-'ohn-ehs)

Chapel
Capilla
(kah-'pee-yah)

Nurse
Enfermero / enfermera
(ehn-fehr-'meh-roh / ehn-fehr-'meh-rah)

Doctor
Doctor / médico / médica
(dohk-'tohr / 'meh-dee-koh / 'meh-dee-kah)

Paramedic
Paramédico
(pah-rah-'meh-dee-koh)

Respiratory therapist
Terapeuta de respiración
(teh-rah-peh-'oo-tah deh rehs-pee-rah-see-'ohn)

Physical therapist
Terapeuta físico
(the-rah-'peh-oo-tah 'fee-see-koh)

Chaplain
Capellán
(kah-peh-'yahn)

7

In the Maternity Ward

8

Birth can be both a joyful and a threatening occasion in the life of a mother and her family. Many Hispanic people have particular cultural or religious beliefs that come into play during labor and delivery of a child. Ask the mother or a family member about them, such as whether a woman in labor wants a specific person with her: *¿Quién le va a acompañar en el parto?* (kee-'ehn leh vah ah ah-kohm-pah-nee-'ahr ehn ehl 'pahr-toh) (*Who is going to be with you during labor?*).

When was the first day of your last ___
¿Cuándo fue el primer día de su último (a) ___
('kwahn-doh fweh ehl pree-'mehr 'dee-ah deh soo 'ool-tee-moh)

Normal menstrual period?
Periodo menstrual normal (regla)?
(peh-ree-'oh-doh mehn-stroo-'ahl nohr-'mahl ('reh-glah))

Have you had surgery ___
¿Ha tenido alguna operación ___? / ¿Le han hecho cirugía ___?
(ah teh-'nee-doh ahl-'goo-nah oh-peh-rah-see-'ohn / leh ahn 'eh-choh see-roo-'hee-ah)

Of the cervix?
Del cuello de la matriz?
(dehl 'kweh-yoh deh lah mah-'trees)

Uterus?
Del útero (matriz)?
(dehl 'oo-teh-roh) (mah-'trees)

Tubal ligation?
De la ligadura de las trompas?
(deh lah lee-gah-'doo-rah deh lahs 'trohm-pahs)

Hysterectomy?
Histerectomía?
(ees-teh-rehk-toh-'mee-ah)

When you were pregnant before,
¿Cuándo estuvo embarazada antes,
('kwahn-doh ehs-'too-boh ehm-bah-rah-'sah-dah 'ahn-tehs)

Did you have
¿Tuvo usted
('too-boh oo-'stehd)

Hypertension?
¿Presión alta?
(preh-see-'ohn 'ahl-tah)

Diabetes?
¿Diabetes?
(dee-ah-'beh-tehs)

Premature labor?
¿Parto (nacimiento) prematuro?
('pahr-toh [nah-see-mee-'ehn-toh] preh-mah-'too-roh)

Postpartum depression?

¿Depresión después del parto?

(deh-preh-see-'ohn dehs-'pwehs dehl 'pahr-toh)

Cesarean section?

¿Cesárea?

(ceh-'sah-ree-ah)

How many times have you been pregnant?

¿Cuántas veces ha estado embarazada?

('kwahn-tahs 'beh-sehs ah ehs-'tah-doh ehm-bah-rah-'sah-dah)

How many miscarriages?

¿Cuántos abortos espontáneos?

('kwahn-tohs ah-'bohr-tohs ehs-pohn-'tah-nee-ohs)

How many abortions?

¿Cuántos abortos provocados?

('kwahn-tohs ah-'bohr-tohs proh-boh-'kah-dohs)

Have you used contraceptives?

¿Ha usado anticonceptivos?

(ah oo-'sah-doh ahn-tee-kohn-sehp-'tee-bohs)

What kind?

¿De qué tipo?

(deh keh 'tee-poh)

When was the last time you took the pills?

¿Cuándo fué la última vez que tomó las píldoras?

('kwahn-doh fweh lah 'ool-tee-mah behs keh toh-'moh lahs 'peel-doh-rahs)

Have you had any bleeding?

¿Ha tenido algún sangrado?

(ah teh-'nee-doh ahl-'goon sahn-'grah-doh)

8

How much?
¿Cuánto?
('kwahn-toh)

Any cramping?
¿Retortijones? (¿Calambres?)
(reh-tohr-tee-'hohn'ehs (kah-'lahm'brehs))

Have you been sick since you got pregnant?
¿Ha estado enferma desde que se embarazó?
(ah ehs-'tah-doh ehn-'fehr-mah' dehs-deh keh seh ehm-bah-rah-'soh)

Any X-rays?
¿Le han tomado rayos X?
(leh ahn toh-'mah-doh 'rah-yohs 'eh-kees)

Any medications?
¿Algún medicamento?
(ahl-'goon meh-dee-kah-'mehn-toh)

Prenatal vitamins?
¿Vitaminas prenatales?
(bee-tah-'mee-nahs preh-nah-'tahl-ehs)

Are your ankles swollen?
¿Se le hinchan los tobillos?
(seh leh 'een-chahn lohs toh-'bee-yohs)

Burning on urination?
¿Le arde cuando orina?
(leh 'ahr-deh 'kwahn-doh oh-'ree-nah)

Frequent urination?
¿Orina frecuentemente?
(oh-'ree-nah freh-kwehn-teh-'mehn-teh)

Blood in your urine?
¿Tiene sangre en la orina?
(tee-'eh-neh 'sahn-greh ehn lah oh-'ree-nah)

Vaginal itching?
¿Comezón vaginal?
(koh-meh-'sohn bah-hee-'nahl)

When did you first notice your baby move?
¿Cuándo notó por primera vez que se movió el bebé?
('kwahn-doh noh-'toh pohr pree-'meh-rah behs keh seh moh-bee-'oh ehl beh-'beh)

How often does he move?
¿Con qué frequencia se mueve?
(kohn keh freh-'kwehn-see-ah seh 'mweh-beh)

Are you going to breast-feed?
¿Va a dar el pecho?
(bah ah dahr ehl 'peh-choh)

Have you ever had ___
¿Ha tenido alguna vez ___
(ah teh-'nee-doh ahl-'goo-nah behs)

Rubella?
¿Rubéola?
(roo-'beh-oh-lah)

Chicken pox?
¿Varicela?
(bah-ree-'seh-lah)

HIV?
¿VIH?
(beh ee 'ah-cheh)

8

Tuberculosis?
¿Tuberculosis?
(too-behr-koo-'loh-sees)

Anemia?
¿Anemia?
(ah-'neh-mee-ah)

Hepatitis?
¿Hepatitis?
(eh-pah-'tee-tees)

➤ *BREAST-FEEDING*

Wash your hands before nursing.
Lávese las manos antes de dar el pecho.
('lah-beh-seh lahs 'mah-nohs 'ahn-tehs deh dahr ehl 'peh-choh)

Wash the nipple with water only, without soap.
Lávese el pezón con agua sin jabón.
('lah-'beh-seh ehl peh-'sohn kohn 'ah-gwah seen hah-'bohn)

You may sit down or lie on the side
Puede sentarse o acostarse del lado
('pweh-deh sehn-'tahr-seh oh ah-koh-'stahr-seh dehl 'lah-doh)

of the breast you are going to feed with
del seno con que va a amamantar
(dehl 'sehn-oh kohn keh bah ah ah-mah-mahn-'tahr)

Hold the baby in your arms.
Sostenga el bebé en sus brazos.
(sohs-'tehn-gah ehl beh-'beh ehn soos 'brah-sohs)

Turn the baby's body toward your breast.
Ponga el bebé contra su pecho.
('pohn-gah ehl beh-'beh 'kohn-trah soo 'peh-choh)

Stroke the baby's cheek with your nipple.
Acaricie la mejilla del bebé con su pezón.
(ah-kah-'ree-see-eh lah meh-'hee-yah dehl beh-'beh kohn soo peh-'sohn)

The baby's mouth should cover
La boca del bebé debe cubrir
(lah 'boh-kah dehl beh-'beh 'deh-beh 'koo-breer)

the whole areola.
toda la aréola.
('toh-dah lah ah-'reh-oh-lah)

Nurse for at least 10 minutes before
Amamante por lo menos diez minutes antes de
(ah-mah-'mahn-teh pohr loh 'meh-nohs 'dee-ehs mee-'noo-tohs 'ahn-tehs deh)

changing breasts.
cambiar del seno.
(deh kahm-bee-'ahr dehl 'sehn-oh)

Never rush feeding.
Nunca de pecho apurada o a la carrera.
('noon-kah deh 'peh-choh ah-poo-'rah-dah oh ah lah kah-'reh-rah)

You should breastfeed every 2 to 3 hours.
Debe amamantar cada dos o tres horas.
('deh-beh ah-mah-mahn-'tahr 'kah-dah dohs oh trehs 'oh-rahs)

8

Burp the baby halfway through feeding
Eructe al bebé a medio comer
(eh-'rook-teh ahl beh-'beh ah 'meh-dee-oh koh-'mehr)

and after feeding.
y después de que ha comido.
(ee dehs-'pwehs deh keh ah koh-'mee-doh)

Wake up the baby by changing the diaper
Despierte al bebé cambiándole pañales
(dehs-pee-'ehr-teh ahl beh-'beh kahm-bee-'ahn-doh-leh pah-'nyah-lehs)

or by rubbing his or her back.
o frotándole la espalda.
(oh frohn-'tahn-doh-leh lah ehs-'pahl-dah)

You may use a breast pump
Puede usar una sacaleche
('pweh-deh oo-'sahr 'oo-nah sah-kah-'leh-cheh)

to pump milk.
para sacar leche.
('pah-rah sah-'kahr 'leh-cheh)

Store each feeding individually.
Almacene cada porción individualmente.
(ahl-mah-'seh-neh 'kah-dah pohr-see-'ohn een-dee-bee-dwal-'mehn-teh)

You may freeze breast milk
Puede congelar la leche de pecho
('pweh-deh kohn-heh-'lahr lah 'leh-cheh deh 'peh-choh)

and thaw it before feeding the baby.
y descongelarla antes de alimentar al bebé.
(ee dehs-kohn-heh-'lahr-lah 'ahn-tehs deh ah-lee-mehn-'tahr ahl beh-'beh)

➤ *BOTTLE FEEDING*

Wash your hands before preparing the formula.
Lávese las manos antes de preparar la fórmula.
('lah-beh-seh lahs 'mah-nohs 'ahn-tehs deh preh-pah-'rahr lah 'fohr-moo-lah)

You may wash bottles and nipples with
Puede lavar las botellas y mamaderas con
('pweh-deh lah-'bahr lahs boh-'teh-yahs ee mah-mah-'deh-rahs kohn)

soap and water.
agua y jabón.
('ah-gwah ee hah-'bohn)

You may prepare feedings individually
Puede preparar porciones individualmente
('pweh-deh preh-pah-'rahr pohr-see-'oh-nehs een-dee-bee-dwahl-'mehn-teh)

or for the entire day.
o para todo el día.
(oh 'pah-rah 'toh-doh ehl 'dee-ah)

You should keep the formula refrigerated.
Debe mantener la fórmula refrigerada.
('deh-beh mahn-teh-'nehr lah 'fohr-moo-lah reh-free-hehr-'rah-dah)

8

You may then warm it before the feeding.
Puede calentarla antes de alimentar al bebé.
(*'pweh-deh kah-lehn-'tahr-lah 'ahn-tehs deh ah-lee-mehn-'tahr ahl beh-'beh*)

Feed your baby every 3 to 4 hours,
Alimente al bebé cada tres o cuatro horas,
(*ah-lee-'mehn-teh ahl beh-'beh 'kah-dah trehs oh 'kwah-troh 'oh-rahs*)

or as the baby requires it.
o cuando el bebé se lo pide.
(*oh koo-'ahn-doh ehl beh-'beh seh loh 'pee-deh*)

Burp your baby frequently.
Eructe al bebé frecuentemente.
(*eh-'rook-teh ahl beh-'beh freh-kwehn-teh-'mehn-teh*)

Do not leave your baby unattended
No deje al bebé desatendido
(*noh 'deh-heh ahl beh-'beh dehs-ah-tehn-'dee-doh*)

when feeding.
cuando esté alimentándolo.
(*'kwahn-doh ehs-'teh ah-lee-mehn-'tahn-doh-loh*)

➤ BATHING

Bathe your baby in warm water.
Bañe al bebé con agua tibia.
(*'bahn-yeh ahl beh-'beh kohn 'ah-gwah 'tee-bee-ah*)

Test the water with your hand
Pruebe el agua con su mano
(*proo-'eh-beh ehl 'ah-gwah kohn soo 'mah-noh*)

8

before bathing the baby
antes de bañar al bebé
('ahn-tehs deh bah-'nyahr ahl beh-'beh)

to make sure it is not too hot.
para asegurarse que no esté muy caliente.
('pah-rah ah-seh-goo-'rahr-seh keh ehs-'teh moo-'ee kah-lee-'ehn-teh)

You can use baby shampoo.
Puede usar champú para bebé.
('pweh-deh 'oo-sahr chahm-'poo 'pah-rah beh-'beh)

Never leave the baby unattended.
Nunca deje al bebé solo.
('noon-kah 'deh-heh ahl beh-'beh 'soh-loh)

You may apply lotion.
Puede ponerle loción.
('pweh-deh pohn-'ehr-leh loh-see-'ohn)

Make sure to dry the baby well.
Asegúrese de secar bien al bebé.
(ah-seh-'goo-reh-seh deh seh-'kahr bee-'ehn ahl beh-'beh)

Make sure to cover the baby right after bathing.
Asegúrese de cubrirlo inmediatemente despues del baño.
(ah-seh-'goo-reh-seh deh koo-'breer-loh een-meh-dee-ah-teh-'mehn-teh dehs-'pwehs dehl 'bah-nyoh)

Do not use cotton swabs to clean
No use palillos con algodón para limpiar
(noh 'oo-seh pah-'lee-yohs kohn ahl-goh-'dohn 'pah-rah leem-pee-'ahr)

8

ears or nose.
los oídos o la nariz.
(lohs oh-'ee-doh oh lah nah-'rees)

➤ *WELL-BABY VISITS*

Make an appointment to see
Haga una cita para ver a
('ah-gah 'oo-nah 'see-tah 'pah-rah behr ah)

your doctor / pediatrician in _____
su doctor / pediatra en _____
(dohk-'tohr / pee-dee-'ah-trah ehn)

two weeks.
dos semanas.
(dohs seh-'mah-nahs)

one month.
un mes.
(oon mehs)

six weeks.
seis semanas.
('seh-ees seh-'mah-nahs)

Your baby got the following vaccinations here:
Su bebé recibió las siguientes vacunas aquí:
(soo beh-'beh reh-see-bee-'oh lahs see-gee-'ehn-tehs bah-'koo-nahs ah-'kee)

Hepatitis B.
Hepatitis B.
(eh-pah-'tee-tees beh)

8

The baby will need the following
El bebe va a necesitar las siguientes
(ehl beh-'beh bah ah neh-seh-'see-tahr lahs see-gee-'ehn-tehs)

vaccinations at
vacunas a los
(bah-'koo-nahs ah lohs)

two and four months:
dos y cuatro meses:
(dohs ee 'kwah-troh 'meh-sehs)

measles-mumps-rubella.
sarampión-paperas-rubéola.
(sah-rahm-pee-'ohn / pah-'peh-rahs / roo-'beh-oh-lah)

polio.
polio.
('poh-lee-oh)

diphtheria-tetanus.
difteria-tétano.
(deef-'teh-ree-ah / 'teh-tah-noh)

pneumococcal vaccine.
vacuna neumocócica.
(bah-'koo-nah neh-oo-moh-'koh-see-kah)

flu vaccine.
vacuna contra la gripe.
(bah-'koo-nah 'kohn-trah lah 'gree-peh)

8

Surgery 9

Many Hispanic, or Latino, people have religious beliefs that the medical practitioner may need to address prior to and after surgery. If the client is Catholic, she or he may request a priest to anoint the sick, or may want to talk to a pastor. *¿Quiere que le llame a un sacerdote?* (*kee-eh-reh keh leh 'yah-meh ah oon sah-sehr-'doh-teh*) (*do you want me to call the priest?*) or *¿Desea una visita del capellán antes de la operación?* (*de-'say-ah 'oon-nah 'vees-'ee-tah dehl cah-peh-'lahn 'ahn-tehs deh lah oh-peh-rah-see-'ohn*) (*do you desire a visit from the chaplain before surgery?*) are questions that may offer the comfort of knowing that you honor the patient's religious beliefs. Sometimes even holding hands in prayer, a smile, or a moment of respectful silence can assist the patient in preparing for surgery.

➤ PREOPERATIVE INSTRUCTIONS

You need to fast after midnight.
Necesita ayunar después de la medianoche.
(*neh-seh-'see-'tah ah-'yoo-'nahr dehs-'pwehs deh lah meh-dee-ah-'noh-cheh*)

Do not have any food or drink after midnight.
No coma, ni tome nada después de la medianoche.
(noh 'koh-mah nee 'toh-meh 'nah-dah dehs-'pwehs deh lah meh-dee-ah-'noh-cheh)

You need to take this medicine.
Necesita tomar esta medicina.
(neh-seh-'see-tah 'toh-mahr 'eh-stah meh-dee-'see-nah)

It is a laxative.
Es un laxante
(ehs oon lahk-'sahn-teh)

I am going to give you an enema.
Le voy a poner una lavativa.
(leh boy ah poh-'nehr 'oo-nah lah-bah-'tee-bah)

You will need someone to pick you up
Va a necesitar que alguien lo recoja
(bah ah neh-seh-see-'tahr keh 'ahl-gee-ehn loh reh-'koh-hah)

after surgery.
después de la cirugía.
(dehs-'pwehs deh lah see-roo-'hee-ah)

Your surgery will take about ___
Su cirugía va a tomar ___
(soo see-roo-'hee-ah bah ah toh-'mahr)

thirty minutes.
treinta minutos.
(treh-'een-tah mee-'noo-tohs)

one hour.
una hora.
('oo-nah 'oh-rah)

9

three hours.
tres horas.
(trehs 'oh-rahs)

You will go to the recovery room after surgery.
Irá a la sala de recuperación después de la cirugía.
(ee-'rah ah lah 'sah-lah deh reh-koo-peh-rah-see-'ohn dehs-'pwehs deh lah see-roo-'hee-ah)

You will be there for a few hours.
Estará allí por unas horas.
(ehs-tah-'rah ah-'yee pohr 'oo-nahs 'oh-rahs)

Your family may wait outside
Su familia puede esperar afuera.
(soo fah-'mee-lee-ah 'pweh-deh ehs-peh-'rahr ah-'fwehr-ah)

We will notify them when the surgery is over.
Les notificaremos cuando termine la cirugía.
(lehs noh-tee-fee-kah-'reh-mohs 'kwahn-doh tehr-'mee-neh lah see-roo-'hee-ah)

Your throat may be sore.
Su garganta le puede doler.
('soo gahr-'gahn-tah leh 'pweh-deh doh-'lehr)

➤ POSTOPERATIVE INSTRUCTIONS

The surgery went well.
La cirugía estuvo bien.
(lah see-roo-'hee-ah 'ehs-'too-boh bee-'ehn)

You will stay here for ___
Va a quedarse aquí por ___
(bah ah keh-'dahr-seh ah-'kee pohr)

9

two hours.
dos horas.
(dohs 'oh-rahs)

four hours.
cuatro horas.
('kwah-troh 'oh-rahs)

We will take you to your room soon.
Le traeremos pronto a su cuarto.
(leh trah-eh-'re-mohs 'prohn-toh 'ah soo 'kwahr-toh')

You will be discharged ___
Será dado de alta ___
(seh-'rah 'dah-doh deh 'ahl-tah)

at noon.
al mediodía.
(meh-dee-oh-'dee-ah)

this afternoon.
esta tarde.
('ehs-tah 'tahr-deh)

this evening.
esta noche.
('ehs-tah 'noh-cheh)

Let me know if you have pain.
Dígame si tiene dolor.
('dee-gah-meh see tee-'eh-neh doh-'lohr)

Let me know if you need to go to the bathroom.
Dígame si necesita ir al baño.
('dee-gah-meh see neh-seh-'see-tah eer ahl 'bahn-'yoh)

9

I will discontinue the Foley in about one hour.
Le voy a quitar su sonda en una hora.
(leh boy ah kee-'tahr soo 'sohn-dah ehn 'oo-nah 'oh-rah)

Cough and take a deep breath.
Tosa y respire profundamente.
('toh-sah ee rehs-'pee-reh proh-foon-dah-'mehn-teh)

Good. Do it again.
Bien. Hágalo de nuevo.
(bee-'ehn 'ah-gah-loh deh 'nweh-boh)

Put this tube in your mouth.
Póngase este tubo en su boca.
('pohn-gah-seh 'ehs-teh 'too-boh ehn soo 'boh-kah)

Take a deep breath.
Respire profundo.
(rehs-'pee-reh proh-'foon-doh)

I am going to leave this spirometer
Le voy a dejar este espirómetro
(leh boy ah deh-'hahr 'ehs-teh ehs-pee-'roh-meh-troh)

at your bedside.
al lado de su cama.
(ahl 'lah-doh deh soo 'kah-mah)

Do these exercises about 10 times every hour.
Haga estos ejercicios como diez veces cada hora.
('ah-gah 'ehs-tohs eh-hehr-see-see-ohs 'koh-moh 'dee-ehs 'beh-sehs 'kah-dah 'oh-rah)

9

➤ DISCHARGE INSTRUCTIONS

Do not change the dressing ___
No cambie el vendaje ___
(noh 'kahm-bee-eh ehl behn-'dah-heh)

until you see your doctor.
hasta que vea a su doctor.
('ahs-tah keh 'beh-ah ah soo dohk-'tohr)

If it gets too drenched,
Si se empapa mucho,
(see seh ehm-'pah-pah 'moo-'choh)

simply add more dressings on top of it.
simplemente agrege más.
(seem-pleh-'mehn-the ah-'greh-geh mahs)

Change the dressing twice a day.
Cambie las gasas dos veces al día.
('kahm-bee-eh lahs 'gah-sahs dohs 'beh-sehs ahl 'dee-ah)

You may only have a liquid diet
Solo puede tomar líquidos claros
('soh-loh 'pweh-deh toh-'mahr 'lee-kee-dohs 'klah-rohs)

until your doctor tells you
hasta que le diga su médico
('ahs-tah keh leh 'dee-gah soo 'meh-dee-koh)

that you can eat other things.
que puede avanzar su dieta.
(keh 'pweh-deh ah-bahn-'sahr soo dee-'eh-tah)

9

Take your medications as instructed.
Tome los medicamentos según las instrucciones.
('toh-meh lohs meh-dee-kah-'mehn-tohs seh-'goon lahs een-strook-see-'ohn-ehs)

You may feel dizzy.
Puede sentirse mareado.
('pweh-deh sehn-'teer-seh mah-reh-'ah-doh)

Do not drive or operate heavy machinery
No maneje ni opere maquinaria pesada
(noh mah-'neh-heh nee oh-'peh-reh mah-kee-'nahr-ee-ah peh-'sah-dah)

while taking these pills.
mientras esté tomando estas pastillas.
(mee-'ehn-trahs ehs-'teh toh-'mahn-doh 'ehs-tahs pah-'stee-yahs)

Call you doctor if you notice
Llame a su doctor si nota
('yah-meh ah soo dohk-'tohr see 'noh-'tah)

excessive bleeding or discharge
sangrado o deshecho excesivo
(sahn-'grah-doh oh dehs-'eh-choh ehk-seh-'see-voh)

from your wound.
de la herida.
(deh lah eh-'ree-dah)

Call 911 if you feel sick.
Llame al nueve uno uno si se siente mal.
('yah-meh ahl 'nweh-beh 'oo-noh 'oo-noh see seh see-'ehn-teh mahl)

9

Glossary

➤ BODY PARTS AND GENERAL VOCABULARY

Abdomen
Abdomen
(ahb-'doh-mehn)

Adam's apple
Manzana de Adán
(mahn-'sah-nah deh ah-'dahn)

Adoption
Adopción
(ah-dohp-see-ohn)

Ankle
Tobillo
(toh-'bee-yoh)

Anus
Ano
('ah-noh)

Arm(s)
Brazo(s)
('brah-soh(s))

Armpit
La axila
(lah ahk-'see-lah)

Artificial limbs and joints
Miembros y coyunturas artificiales
(mee-'em-brohs ee coh-yoon-'too-rahs ar-tee-fee-see-'ah-lehs)

Back
Espalda
(ehs-'pahl-dah)

Backaches
Dolores de espalda
(doh-'loh-rehs deh ehs-'pahl-dah)

Band-Aid
Curita
(koo-'ree-tah)

Bassinet
El bacinete
(ehl bah-see-'neh-teh)

Belly button
Ombligo
(ohm-'blee-goh)

Biceps
Bíceps
('bee-sehps)

Glossary

Blanket
La cobija
(lah koh-`bee-hah)

Blocked artery
La arteria obstruida
(lah ahr-`teh-ree-ah ohb-stroo-`ee-dah)

Breast
Pecho
('peh-choh)

Breathe
Aliento
(ah-lee-`ehn-toh)

Buttocks
Sentaderas / nalgas
(sehn-tah-'deh-rahs/'nahl-gahs)

Calf
Pantorrilla
(pahn-toh-'ree-yah)

Cervical canal
Canal cervical
(kah-`nahl sehr-bee-`kahl)

Cervix
Cuello uterino
('kweh-yoh oo-teh-`ree-noh)

Cheek
Mejilla
(meh-'hee-yah)

Chest
Pecho
(*'peh-choh*)

Chin
Barbilla
(*bahr-'bee-yah*)

Clitoris
Clítoris
(*'klee-toh-rees*)

Collarbone
La clavícula
(*lah klah-'bee-koo-lah*)

Colon
El colon
(*ehl koh-'lohn*)

Diaphragm
Diafragma
(*dee-ah-'frahg-mah*)

Dislocated shoulder
Hombro dislocado
(*'ohm-broh dees-loh-'kah-doh*)

Double vision
Visión doble
(*'bee-see-ohn doh-bleh*)

Ear
Oído
(*oh-'ee-doh*)

Elbow
Codo
('koh-doh)

Embryo
Embrión
(ehm-bree-'ohn)

Esophagus
Esófago
(eh-'soh-fah-goh)

External oblique
Oblicuo mayor
(oh-'blee-koo-oh mah-'yohr)

Extremities
Extremidades
(eks-treh-mee-'dah-dehs)

Eye
Ojo
('oh-hoh)

Face
Cara
('kah-rah)

Fallopian tubes
Trompas de Falopio
('trohm-pahs deh fah-'loh-pee-oh)

Feminine napkin
El paño higiénico
(ehl 'pah-nyoh ee-hee-'eh-nee-koh)

Fertilization
La fertilización
(lah fehr-tee-lee-sah-see-'ohn)

Finger
Dedo
('deh-doh)

Folic acid
Ácido fólico
('ah-see-doh 'foh-lee-koh)

Foot
Pie
(pee-'eh)

Forehead
Frente
('frehn-teh)

German measles
Rubéola
(roo-`beh-oh-lah)

Groin
La ingle
(lah `een-gleh)

Hair
Pelo
('peh-loh)

Hand
Mano
('mah-noh)

Head
Cabeza
(kah-'beh-sah)

Heart Murmur
Murmullos en el corazón
(moor-'moo-yohs ehn ehl koh-rah-'sohn)

Heel
Talón
(tah-'lohn)

Hip
Cadera
(kah-'deh-rah)

Hypertension
Hipertensión
(ee-pehr-tehn-see-'ohn)

Immunotherapy
inmunoterapia
(een-moo-noh-teh-'rah-pee-ah)

Impacted tooth
diente impactado
(dee-'ehn-teh eem-pahk-'tah-doh)

Index finger
Dedo índice
('deh-doh 'een-dee-seh)

Infant car seat
el asiento para infantes
(ehl ah-see-'ehn-toh 'pah-rah een-'fahn-tehs)

Inflammation
Inflamación
(een-flah-mah-see-`ohn)

Ingrown toenail
Uña encarnada
(´oo-nyah ehn-kahr-`nah-dah)

Insanity
Locura
(loh-`koo-rah)

Insect bite
Mordedura de insecto
(mohr-deh-`doo-rah deh een-`sehk-toh)

Intermittent
Intermitente
(een-tehr-mee-`tehn-teh)

Intoxication
Intoxicación
(een-tohk-see-kah-see-ohn)

Jaw
Mandíbula
(mahn-´dee-boo-lah)

Knee
Rodilla
(roh-´dee-yah)

Kneecap
la rótula
(lah `roh-too-lah)

Large Intestine
Intestino grueso
(een-tehs-`tee-noh groo-`eh-soh) .

Larynx
Laringe
(lah-'reen-heh)

Leg
Pierna
(pee-'ehr-nah)

Little finger
Meñique
(meh-'nyee-keh)

Low blood pressure
Presión baja
(preh-see-`ohn 'ba-ha)

Lozenge
Pastilla
(pahs-`tee-yah)

Mastectomy
Mastectomía
(mahs-tehk-toh-`mee-ah)

Maternity Ward
Sala de maternidad
(`sah-lah deh mah-tehr-nee-`dahd)

Measles
Sarampión
(sah-rahm-pee-'ohn)

Meningitis
Meningitis
(meh-neen-`hee-tees)

Menstrual cycle
Ciclo menstrual
(seek-loh mehn-stroo-`ahl)

Mental illness
Enfermedad mental
(ehn-fehr-meh-`dahd mehn-`tahl)

Middle finger
Dedo cordial / dedo de en medio
('deh-doh kohr-dee-'ahl / 'deh-doh deh ehn 'meh-dee-oh)

Morphine
Morfina
(mohr-`fee-nah)

Mouth
Boca
('boh-kah)

Muscle
Músculo
('moos-koo-loh)

Nails
Uñas
('oon-yahs)

Near-sighted
Miope
(mee-`oh-peh)

Neck
Cuello
('kweh-yoh)

Nose
Nariz
(nah-'rees)

Numbness
Adormecimiento
(ah-dohr-meh-see-mee-'ehn-toh)

Nutrition
Nutrición
(noo-tree-see-'ohn)

Ovary
Ovario
(oh-'bah-ree-oh)

Palm
La palma de la mano
(lah 'pahl-mah deh lah 'mah-noh)

Palpitation
palpitación
(pahl-pee-tah-see-'ohn)

Pelvic infection
Infección pélvica
(een-fex-see-'oh 'pehl-bee-kah)

Penis
Pene
('peh-neh)

Peroneus
Peroneo largo
(peh-roh-`neh-oh `lahr-goh)

Potassium
potasio
(poh-`tah-see-oh)

Prostate
Próstata
('prohs-tah-tah)

Psychiatric hospital
Hospital psiquiátrico
(ohs-pee-`tahl see-kee-`aht-ree-koh)

Radiation therapy
Radioterapia
(rah-dee-oh-teh-`rah-pee-ah)

Reconstruction
Reconstrucción
(reh-kohns-trook-see-`ohn)

Rectum
Recto
(rehk-toh)

Rehabilitation
Rehabilitación
(reh-ah-bee-lee-tah-see-`ohn)

Ribcage
Costillas
(kohs-'tee-yahs)

Ring finger
Dedo anular
('deh-doh ah-noo-'lahr)

Scrotum
Escroto
(ehs-'kroh-toh)

Sex organs
Órganos sexuales
('ohr-gah-nohs sehk-soo-'ah-lehs)

Shellfish
mariscos
(mah-`rees-kohs)

Shoulders
Hombros
('ohm-brohs)

Skeleton
esqueleto
(ehs-keh-'leh-toh)

Skin
Piel
(pee-'ehl)

Skull
Cráneo
('krah-nee-oh)

Sleeve
manga
('mahn-gah)

Small Intestine
Intestino Delgado
(een-tehs-`tee-noh dehl-`gah-doh)

Sole
La planta de pie
(lah `plahn-tah dehl pee-`eh)

Spinal cord
Médula espinal
('meh-doo-lah ehs-pee-'nahl)

Spine
Espina dorsal
(ehs-'pee-nah dohr-'sahl)

Stethoscope
Estetoscopio
(ehs-teh-toh-`skoh-pee-oh)

Stillborn
Nacido muerto
(nah-`see-doh 'mwehr-toh)

Straight Jacket
Camisa de fuerza
(kah-`mee-sah deh 'fwehr-sah)

Strangulation
Estrangulamiento
(ehs-trahn-goo-lah-mee-`ehn-toh)

Teeth
Dientes
(dee-'ehn-tehs)

Testicle
Testículo
(tehs-'tee-koo-loh)

Thigh
Muslo
('moos-loh)

Throat
Garganta
(gahr-'gahn-tah)

Thumb
Pulgar
(pool-'gahr)

Toe
Dedo del pie
('deh-doh dehl pee-'eh)

Tongue
Lengua
('lehn-gwah)

Tonsils
Amígdalas
(ah'meeg-dah-lahs)

Torso
Torso
('tohr-soh)

Transfusion
Transfusion
(trahns-foo-see-`ohn)

Trapezius
trapecio
(trah-`peh-see-oh)

Triceps
Tríceps
('tree-sehps)

Uterus
Útero / matriz
('oo-teh-roh / mah-'trees)

Vagina
Vagina
(bah-'hee-nah)

Water Fountain
fuente de agua
('fwehn-teh deh 'ah-gwah)

Wheeze
Silbido
(seel-'bee-do)

Worms
Lombrices
(lohm-'bree-sehs)

Wrist
Muñeca
(moo-'nyeh-kah)

➤ *ORGANS AND SYSTEMS*

Appendix
Apéndice
(ah-'pehn-dee-seh)

Arteries
Arterias
(ahr-'teh-ree-ahs)

Arterioles
Arteriolas
(ahr-teh-ree-'oh-lahs)

Atrium
Aurícula
(ah-oo-'ree-koo-lah)

Bladder
Vejiga
(beh-'hee-gah)

Brain
Cerebro
(seh-'reh-broh)

Brainstem
Tronco cerebral
('trohn-koh seh-reh-'brahl)

Bronchi
Bronquios
('brohn-kee-ohs)

Bronchioles
Bronquiolos
(brohn-kee-'oh-lohs)

Capillary
Capilar
(kah-pee-'lahr)

Cardiovascular system
Aparato cardiovascular
(ah-pah-'rah-toh kahr-dee-oh-bahs-koo-'lahr)

Cerebellum
Cerebelo
(seh-reh-'beh-loh)

Cerebral cortex
Corteza cerebral
(kohr-'teh-sah seh-reh-'brahl)

Circulatory system
Aparato circulatorio
(ah-pah-'rah-toh seer-koo-lah-'toh-ree-oh)

Endocrine system
Sistema endocrino
(sees-'teh-mah ehn-doh-'kree-noh)

Gallbladder
Vesícula biliar
(beh-'see-koo-lah bee-lee-'ahr)

Gastrointestinal system
Sistema digestivo / gastrointestinal
(sees-'teh-mah dee-hehs-'tee-voh / gahs-troh-een-tehs-tee-'nahl)

Heart
Corazón
(koh-rah-'sohn)

Hypothalamus
Hipotálamo
(ee-poh-'tah-lah-moh)

Kidneys
Riñones
(ree-'nyohn-ehs)

Liver
Hígado
('ee-gah-doh)

Lungs
Pulmones
(pool-'mohn-ehs)

Lymphatic system
Sistema linfático
(sees-'teh-mah leen-'fah-tee-koh)

Medulla
Médula
('meh-doo-lah)

Musculoskeletal system
Sistema músculoesquelético
(sees-'teh-mah moos-koo-loh-ehs-keh-'leh-tee-koh)

Nervous system
Sistema nervioso
(sees-'teh-mah nehr-bee-'oh-soh)

Pancreas
Páncreas
('pahn-kreh-ahs)

Parathyroids
Glándulas paratiroides
('glahn-doo-lahs pah-rah-tee-'roh-ee-dehs)

Pituitary gland
Glándula pituitaria
('glahn-doo-lah pee-too-ee-'tah-ree-ah)

Pons
Pons
(pohns)

Pupil(s)
Pupila(s)
(poo-'pee-lah(s))

Respiratory system
Sistema respiratorio
(sees-'teh-mah rehs-pee-rah-'toh-ree-oh)

Sinuses
Senos
('seh-nohs)

Spleen
Bazo
('bah-soh)

Stomach
Estómago
(ehs-'toh-mah-goh)

Thymus
Timo
('tee-moh)

Thyroid
Glándula tiroides
('glahn-doo-lah tee-'roh-ee-dehs)

Tympanic membrane
Membrana del tímpano
(mehm-'brah-nah dehl 'teem-pah-noh)

Ureter(s)
Uréter(es)
(oo-'reh-tehr/tehres)

Urethra
Uretra
(oo-'reh-trah)

Urinary system
Sistema urinario
(sees-'teh-mah oo-ree-'nah-ree-oh)

Valve(s)
Válvula(s)
('bahl-boo-lah(s))

Veins
Venas
('beh-nahs)

Ventricle
Ventrículo
(behn-'tree-koo-loh)

➤ *COMMON ILLNESSES BY SYSTEM*

Head, Eye, Ear, Nose, and Throat

Acute otitis
Otitis aguda
(oh-'tee-tees ah-'goo-dah)

Allergic conjunctivitis
Conjuntivitis alérgica
('kohn-hoon-tee-'bee-tees ah-'lehr-hee-kah)

Allergic rhinitis
Rinitis alérgica
(ree-'nee-tees ah-'lehr-hee-kah)

Astigmatism
Astigmatismo
(ah-steeg-mah-'tees-moh)

Blepharitis
Blefaritis
(bleh-fah-'ree-tees)

Cataracts
Cataratas
(kah-tah-'rah-tahs)

Chalazion
Chalazión / calacio
(chah-lah-see-'ohn / kah-'lah-see-oh)

Conjunctivitis
Conjuntiviti
(kohn-hoon-tee-'bee-tees)

Cornea laceration
Laceración de la cornea
(lah-sehr-rah-see-'ohn deh lah 'kohr-neh-ah)

Deafness
Sordera
(sohr-'deh-rah)

Deviated septum
Desviación septal
(dehs-bee-ah-see-'ohn sehp-'tahl)

Diabetic retinopathy
Retinopatía diabetica
(reh-tee-noh-pah-'tee-ah dee-ah-'beh-tee-kah)

Ear infection
Infección del oído
(een-fehk-see-'ohn dehl oh-'ee-doh)

Epistaxis
Sangrado de nariz / Epistaxis
(sahn-'grah-doh deh nah-'rees / eh-pees-'tahk-sees)

External otitis
Otitis externa
(oh-'tee-tees ehks-'tehr-nah)

Eye infection
Infección del ojo
(een-fehk-see-'ohn dehl 'oh-hoh)

Glaucoma
Glaucoma
(glaw-'koh-mah)

Headache
Dolor de cabeza
(doh-'lohr deh kah-'beh-sah)

Hordeolum
Orzuelo
(or-'sweh-loh)

Hyperopia
Hipermetropía / hiperopía
(ee-pehr-meh-troh-'pee-ah / ee-peh-ro-'pee-ah)

Influenza
Influenza
(een-floo-'ehn-sah)

Labyrinthitis
Laberentitis
(lah-behr-ehn-'tee-tees)

Laryngitis
Laringitis
(lah-reen-'hee-tees)

Loss of hearing
Pérdida del oído
('pehr-dee-dah dehl oh-'ee-doh)

Macular degeneration
Degeneración macular
(deh-heh-neh-rah-see-'ohn mah-koo-'lahr)

Meniere's disease
Enfermedad de Meniere
(ehn-fehr-meh-'dahd deh mehn-ee-'eh-reh)

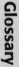

Glossary

Myopia
Miopía
(mee-oh-'pee-ah)

Pharyngitis
Faringitis
(fah-reen-'hee-tees)

Retinal detachment
Separación de la retina
(seh-pah-rah-see-'ohn deh lah reh-'tee-nah)

Rhinitis
Rinitis
(ree-'nee-tees)

Runny nose
Nariz congestionada
(nah-'rees kohn-hehs-tee-oh-'nah-dah)

Ruptured tympanic membrane
Tímpano roto
('teem-pah-noh 'roh-toh)

Sinusitis
Sinusitis
(see-noo-'see-tees)

Sore throat
Dolor de garganta
(doh-'lohr deh gahr-'gahn-tah)

Strabismus
Estrabismo
(ehs-trah-'bees-moh)

Tonsillitis
Amigdalitis
(ah-meeg-dah-'lee-tees)

Respiratory

Acute bronchitis
Bronquitis aguda
(brohn-'kee-tees ah-'goo-dah)

Apnea
Apnea
('ahp-neh-ah)

Asthma
Asma
('ahs-mah)

Atelectasis
Atelactasia
(ah-teh-lahk-'tah-see-ah)

Bronchitis
Bronquitis
(brohn-'kee-tees)

Cancer of the larynx
Cáncer de la laringe
('kahn-sehr deh lah lah-'reen-heh)

Chronic bronchitis
Bronquitis crónica
(brohn-'kee-tees 'kroh-nee-kah)

Chronic obstructive pulmonary disease
Enfermedad crónica pulmonar
(ehn-fehr-meh-'dahd 'kroh-nee-kah pool-moh-'nahr)

Emphysema
Enfisema
(ehn-fee-'seh-mah)

Influenza
Influenza
(een-floo-'ehn-sah)

Lung cancer
Cáncer del pulmón
('kahn-sehr del pool-'mohn)

Pleural effusion
Hidrotórax
(ee-droh-'toh-rahks)

Pleurisy
Pleuresía
(pleh-oo-reh-'see-ah)

Pneumonia
Neumonía
(neh-oo-'moh-'nee-ah)

Pneumothorax
Neumotórax
(neh-oo-moh-'toh-rahks)

Pulmonary edema
Edema pulmonar
(eh-'deh-mah pool-moh-'nahr)

Pulmonary embolus
Embolia pulmonar
(ehm-'boh-lee-ah pool-moh-'nahr)

Severe acute respiratory syndrome (SARS)
Síndrome agudo del aparato respiratorio
*('seen-droh-meh ah-'goo-doh dehl ah-pah-'rah-toh rehs-pee-rah-
'toh-ree-oh)*

Tuberculosis
Tuberculosis
(too-behr-koo-'loh-sees)

Upper airway obstruction
Obstrucción de las vías respiratorias superiores
*(ohb-strook-see-'ohn deh lahs 'bee-ahs rehs-pee-rah-'toh-ree-ahs
soo-peh-ree-'oh-rehs)*

Cardiovascular / Peripheral Vascular

Angina
Angina del pecho
(ahn-'hee-nah dehl 'peh-choh)

Arterial aneurysm
Aneurisma arterial
(ah-neh-oo-'rees-mah ahr-teh-ree-'ahl)

Arterial embolism
Embolismo arterial
(ehm-boh-'lees-moh ahr-teh-ree-'ahl)

Arteriosclerosis
Arteriosclerosis
(ahr-teh-ree-oh-skleh-'roh-sees)

Atherosclerosis
Aterosclerosis
(ah-teh-roh-skleh-'roh-sees)

Atrial fibrillation
Fibrilación auricular
(fee-bree-lah-see-'ohn ah-oo-ree-koo-'lahr)

Atrioventricular block
Bloqueo atrioventricular
(bloh-'keh-oh ah-tree-oh-behn-tree-koo-'lahr)

Cardiogenic shock
Choque cardiogénico
('cho-keh kahr-dee-oh-'heh-nee-koh)

Cardiomyopathy
Cardiomiopatía
(kahr-dee-oh-mee-oh-pah-'tee-ah)

Deep venous thrombosis
Trombosis venosa profunda
(trohm-'boh-sees beh-'noh-sah proh-'foon-dah)

Fat embolism
Embolia de grasa
(ehm-'boh-lee-ah deh 'grah-sah)

Heart attack
Ataque al corazón
(ah-'tah-keh ahl koh-rah-'sohn)

Heart failure (congestive)
Insuficiencia cardiaca (congestiva)
(een-soo-fee-see-'ehn-see-ah kahr-'dee-ah-kah (kohn-heh-'stee-bah))

High blood pressure
Presión alta
(preh-see-'ohn 'ahl-tah)

Hyperlipidimia
Hiperlipidemia
(ee-pehr-lee-pee-'deh-mee-ah)

Hypertension
Hipertensión
(ee-per-ten-see-ohn)

Myocardial infarction
Infarto del miocardio
(een-'fahr-toh dehl mee-oh-'kahr-dee-oh)

Myocarditis
Miocarditis
(mee-oh-kahr-'dee-tees)

Pericarditis
Pericarditis
(peh-ree-kahr-'dee-tees)

Premature ventricular *contractions (PVC)*
Extrasistoles
(ehks-trah-see-'stoh-lehs)

Raynaud's disease
Enfermedad de Raynaud
(ehn-fehr-meh-'dahd deh ray-'nah-ood)

Rheumatic fever
Fiebre reumática
(fee-'eh-breh reh-oo-'mah-tee-kah)

Sinus bradycardia
Bradicardia sinusal
(brah-dee-'kahr-dee-ah see-noo-'sahl)

Sinus tachycardia
Taquicardia sinusal
(tah-kee-'kahr-dee-ah see-noo-'sahl)

Supraventricular tachycardia
Taquicardia supraventricular
(tah-kee-'kahr-dee-ah soo-prah-behn-tree-koo-'lahr)

Thromboembolus
Tromboembolismo
(trohm-boh-ehm-boh-'lees-moh)

Thrombophlebitis
Tromboflebitis
(trohm-boh-fleh-'bee-tees)

Valvular heart disease
Enfermedad cardiaca valvular
(ehn-fehr-meh-'dahd kahr-'dee-ah-kah bahl-boo-'lahr)

Varicose veins
Venas varicosas
('beh-nahs bah-ree-'koh-sahs)

Venous stasis ulcers
Úlceras por insuficiencia venosa
('ool-seh-rahs pohr een-soo-fee-see-'ehn-see-ah beh-'noh-sah)

Ventricular tachycardia
Taquicardia ventricular
(tah-kee-'kahr-dee-ah behn-tree-koo-'lahr)

Glossary

Gastrointestinal

Anal fissure
Fisura anal
(fee-'soo-rah ah-'nahl)

Anal fistula
Fístula anal
('fees-too-lah ah-'nahl)

Anorexia
Anorexia
(ah-noh-'rehk-see-ah)

Appendicitis
Apendicitis
(ah-pehn-dee-'see-tees)

Ascites
Ascitis
(ah-'see-tees)

Bowel (fecal) incontinence
Incontinencia fecal
(een-kohn-tee-'nehn-see-ah feh-'kahl)

Cancer of the pancreas
Cáncer del páncreas
('kahn-sehr dehl 'pahn-kree-ahs)

Carcinoma of the liver
Carcinoma del hígado
(kahr-see-'noh-mah dehl 'ee-gah-doh)

Carcinoma of the mouth
Carcinoma de la boca
(kahr-see-'noh-mah deh lah 'boh-kah)

Cavities (dental cavities)
Cavidades (caries dentales)
(kah-bee-'dah-dehs ('kah-ree-ehs dehn-'tahl-ehs))

Cirrhosis
Cirrosis
(see-'roh-sees)

Colitis
Colitis
(koh-'lee-tees)

Colon cancer
Cáncer del colon
('kahn-sehr dehl 'koh-lohn)

Constipation
Constipación / estreñimiento
(kohn-stee-pah-see-'ohn / ehs-treh-nyee-mee-'ehn-toh)

Crohn's disease
Enfermedad de Crohn
(ehn-fehr-meh-'dahd deh krohn)

Dental plaque
Placa dental
('plah-kah dehn-'tahl)

Diarrhea
Diarrhea
(dee-ah-'rreh-ah)

Diverticulitis
Diverticulitis
(dee-behr-tee-koo-'lee-tees)

Duodenal ulcer
Úlcera duodenal
('ool-seh-rah doo-oh-deh-'nahl)

Esophageal varices
Varices del esófago
(bah-'ree-sehs dehl eh-'soh-fah-goh)

Gallstones
Piedras en la vesicula
(pee-'eh-drahs ehn lah beh-'see-koo-lah)

Gastric ulcer
Úlcera gástrica
('ool-seh-rah 'gahs-tree-kah)

Gastritis
Gastritis
(gahs-'tree-tees)

Gastroesophageal reflux
Reflujo gastroesofágico
(reh-'floo-hoh gahs-troh-eh-soh-'fah-hee-koh)

Hemorrhoids
Hemorroides
(eh-moh-'rroh-ee-dehs)

Hepatic encephalopathy
Encefalopatía hepática
(ehn-seh-fah-loh-pah-'tee-ah eh-'pah-tee-kah)

Hepatitis
Hepatitis
(eh-pah-'tee-tees)

Hernia
Hernia
('ehr-nee-ah)

Hiatal hernia
Hernia hiatal
('ehr-nee-ah ee-ah-'tahl)

Irritable bowel syndrome
Síndrome de colon irritable
('seen-droh-meh deh koh-'lohn ee-ree-'tah-bleh)

Liver abscess
Abceso hepático
(ahb-'seh-soh eh-'pah-tee-koh)

Malaria
Malaria (Paludismo)
(mah-`lah-ree-ah)

Oral candidiasis
Candidiasis oral
(kahn-dee-dee-'ah-sees oh-'rahl)

Peptic ulcer
Úlcera péptica
('ool-seh-rah 'pehp-tee-kah)

Peritonitis
Peritonitis
(peh-ree-toh-'nee-tees)

Stomach infection
Infección del estómago
(een-fehk-see-'ohn dehl ehs-'toh-mah-goh)

Urinary / Genital

Benign prostatic hypertrophy
Hipertrofia prostática benigna
(ee-pehr-troh-'fee-ah proh-'stah-tee-kah beh-'neeg-nah)

Cancer of the prostate
Cáncer de la próstata
('kahn-sehr deh lah 'pros-tah-tah)

Chronic renal failure
Insuficiencia renal crónica
(een-soo-fee-see-'ehn-see-ah reh-'nahl 'kroh-nee-kah)

Cystitis
Cistitis
(sees-'tee-tees)

Gonorrhea
Gonorrea
(goh-noh-`rreh-ah)

Hydronephrosis
Hidronefrosis
(ee-droh-neh-'froh-sees)

Kidney stones
Piedras en el riñón
(pee-'eh-drahs ehn ehl ree-nee-'ohn)

Nephritis
Nefritis
(neh-'free-tees)

Nephrotic syndrome
Síndrome nefrótico
('seen-droh-meh neh-'froh-tee-koh)

Prostatitis
Prostatitis
(prohs-tah-'tee-tees)

Pyelonephritis
Pielonefritis
(pee-ehl-oh-neh-'free-tees)

Renal failure
Insuficiencia renal
(een-soo-fee-see-'ehn-see-ah reh-'nahl)

Syphilis
Sífilis
('see-fee-lees)

Tumor of the bladder
Tumor de la vejiga
(too-'mohr deh lah beh-'hee-gah)

Tumor of the kidney
Tumor del riñón
(too-'mohr dehl rene-'yohn)

Urethritis
Uretritis
(oo-reh-'tree-tees)

Urinary obstruction
Obstrucción de las vías urinarias
(ohb-strohk-see-'ohn deh lahs 'bee-ahs oo-ree-'nah-ree-ahs)

Venereal disease
Enfermedad venerea
(ehn-fehr-meh-`dahd beh-`neh-reh-ahl)

Musculoskeletal

Amputation
Amputación
(ahm-poo-tah-see-'ohn)

Ankle sprain
Torcedura del tobillo
(tohr-seh-'doo-rah dehl toh-'bee-yoh)

Arthritis
Artritis
(ahr-'tree-tees)

Bone tumor
Tumor de hueso
(too-'mohr deh 'weh-soh)

Carpal tunnel syndrome
Síndrome del canal del carpo
('seen-droh-meh dehl kah-'nahl dehl 'kahr-poh)

Contusion
Contusión
(kohn-too-see-'ohn)

Dislocation
Luxación
(loohks-ah-see-'ohn)

Fracture
Fractura
(frahk-'too-rah)

Fracture of the arm
Fractura del brazo
(frahk-'too-rah dehl 'brah-soh)

Fracture of the back
Fractura de la espalda
(frahk-'too-rah deh lah ehs-'pahl-dah)

Fracture of the foot
Fractura del pie
(frahk-'too-rah dehl pee-'eh)

Fracture of the hand
Fractura de la mano
(frahk-'too-rah deh lah 'mah-noh)

Fracture of the hip
Fractura de la cadera
(frahk-'too-rah deh lah kah-'deh-rah)

Fracture of the leg
Fractura de la pierna
(frahk-'too-rah deh lah pee-'ehr-nah)

Fracture of the pelvis
Fractura de la pelvis
(frahk-'too-rah deh lah 'pehl-bees)

Gout
Gota
('goh-tah)

Herniated disk
Disco herniado
('dees-koh ehr-nee-'ah-doh)

Muscular dystrophy
distrofia muscular
(dees-'troh-fee-ah moos-koo-'lahr)

Osteoarthritis
Osteoarthritis
(oh-stee-oh-ahr-'tree-tees)

Osteomyelitis
Osteomielitis
(oh-stee-oh-mee-eh-'lee-tees)

Osteoporosis
Osteoporosis
(oh-stee-oh-poh-'roh-sees)

Rheumatoid arthritis
Artritis reumática
(ahr-'tree-tees reh-oo-'mah-tee-kah)

Strain
Torcedura
(tohr-seh-'doo-rah)

Whiplash lesion
Lesion de latigazo
(leh-see-'ohn deh lah-tee-'gah-soh)

Hematologic / Lymphatic

Acquired immunodeficiency syndrome (AIDS)
Síndrome de inmunodeficiencia adquirida (SIDA)
('seen-droh-meh deh een-moo-noh-deh-fee-see-'ehn-see-ah ahd-kee-'ree-dah ('eh-seh ee deh ah))

Anemia
Anemia
(ah-'neh-mee-ah)

Aplastic anemia
Anemia aplástica
(ah-'neh-mee-ah ah-'plahs-tee-kah)

Gangrene
Gangrena
(gahn-greh-nah)

Hemophilia
Hemofilia
(eh-moh-'fee-lee-ah)

Hemorrhoids
Hemorroides
(eh-moh-`rroh-ee-dehs)

Hemorrhage
Hemorragia
(eh-mohr-`rah-hee-ah)

Hodgkin's disease
Enfermedad de Hodgkin
(ehn-fehr-meh-'dahd deh hodgkin)

Hospitalization
Hospitalización
(ohs-pee-tah-lee-sah-see-ohn)

Human immunodeficiency virus (HIV)
Virus de inmunodeficiencia humano (VIH)
('bee-roos deh een-moo-noh-deh-fee-see-'ehn-see-ah oo-'mah-noh)

Hydrogen peroxide
Agua oxigenada
(ah-gwah ohk-see-heh-`nah-dah)

Glossary

Iron-deficiency anemia
Anemia de deficiencia de hierro
(ah-'neh-mee-ah deh deh-fee-see-'ehn-see-ah deh 'yeh-roh)

Leukemia
Leucemia
(leh-oo-'seh-mee-ah)

Multiple myeloma
Mieloma múltiple
(mee-eh-'loh-mah 'mool-tee-pleh)

Non-Hodgkin's lymphoma
Limfoma non-Hodgkin
(leem-'foh-mah nohn-hodgkin)

Pernicious anemia
Anemia perniciosa
(ah-'neh-mee-ah pehr-nee-see-'oh-sah)

Sickle-cell anemia
Anemia falciforme / drepanocítica
(ah-'neh-mee-ah fahl-see-'fohr-meh / dreh-pah-noh-'see-tee-kah)

Endocrine

Acromegaly
Acromegalia
(ah-kroh-meh-'gah-lee-ah)

Addison's disease
Enfermedad de Addison
(ehn-fehr-meh-'dahd deh addison)

Glossary

Cancer of the thyroid
Cáncer de la glándula tiroides
('kahn-sehr deh lah 'glahn-doo-lah tee-'roh-ee-dehs)

Cushing's syndrome
Síndrome de Cushing
('seen-droh-meh deh cushing)

Diabetes
Diabetes
(dee-ah-'beh-tehs)

Dwarfism
Enanismo
(eh-nah-'nees-moh)

Gigantism
Gigantismo
(hee-gahn-'tees-moh)

Goiter
Bocio
('boh-see-oh)

Graves' Disease
Enfermedad de Graves
(ehn-fehr-meh-'dahd deh graves)

Hyperparathyroidism
Hiperparatiroidismo
(ee-pehr-pah-rah-tee-roh-ee-'dees-moh)

Hyperthyroidism
Hipertiroidismo
(ee-pehr-tee-roh-ee-'dees-moh)

Glossary

Hypoparathyroidism
Hipoparatiroidismo
(ee-poh-pah-rah-tee-roh-ee-'dees-moh)

Hypothyroidism
Hipotiroidismo
(ee-poh-tee-roh-'dees-moh)

Neurologic

Alzheimer's disease
Enfermedad de Alzheimer
(ehn-fehr-meh-'dahd deh alzheimer)

Bell's palsy
Parálisis de Bell
(pah-'rah-lee-sees deh bell)

Craniocerebral trauma
Trauma craniocerebral
('trah-oo-mah krah-nee-oh-seh-reh-'brahl)

Epilepsy
Epilepsia
(eh-pee-'lehp-see-ah)

Guillain-Barré syndrome
Síndrome de Guillain-Barré
('seen-droh-meh deh guillian-barré)

Headache
Dolor de cabeza
(doh-'lohr deh kah-'beh-sah)

Huntington's disease
Enfermedad de Huntington
(ehn-fehr-meh-'dahd deh huntington)

Increased intercranial pressure
Presión intercraneal elevada
(preh-see-'ohn een-tehr-krah-neh-'ahl eh-leh-'bah-dah)

Multiple sclerosis
Esclerosis múltiple
(ehs-kleh-'roh-sees 'mool-tee-pleh)

Myasthenia gravis
Miastenia gravis
(mee-ahs-'teh-nee-ah 'grah-bees)

Parkinson's disease
Enfermedad de Parkinson
(ehn-fehr-meh-'dahd deh 'parh-keen-sohn)

Seizures
Convulsiones
(kohn-vool-see-'oh-nehs)

Spinal cord trauma
Trauma de la médula espinal
('trah-oo-mah deh lah 'meh-doo-lah ehs-pee-'nahl)

Stroke
Embolia
(ehm-'boh-lee-ah)

Trigeminal neuralgia
Neuralgia trigeminal
(neh-oo-'rahl-hee-ah tree-heh-mee-nahl)

Glossary

Dermatologic

Acne
Acné
(ahk-'neh)

Alopecia
Alopecia
(ah-loh-'peh-see-ah)

Burns
Quemaduras
(keh-mah-'doo-rahs)

First-degree burn
Quemadura de primer grado
(keh-mah-'doo-rah deh pree-'mehr 'grah-doh)

Full thickness burn
Quemadura total
(keh-mah-'doo-rah toh-'tahl)

Lice
Piojos
(pee-'oh-hohs)

Partial thickness burn
Quemadura parcial
(keh-mah-'doo-rah pahr-see-'ahl)

Second-degree burn
Quemadura de segundo grado
(keh-mah-'doo-rah deh seh-'goon-doh 'grah-'doh)

Superficial burn
Quemadura superficial
(keh-mah-'doo-rah soo-pehr-fee-see-'ahl)

Third-degree burn
Quemadura de tercer grado
(keh-mah-'doo-rah deh tehr-'sehr 'grah-doh)

Cellulitis
Celulitis
(seh-loo-'lee-tees)

Contact dermatitis
Dermatitis de contacto
(dehr-mah-'tees-tees deh kohn-'tahk-toh)

Eczema
Eczema
(ehk-'seh-mah)

Folliculitis
Foliculitis
(foh-lee-koo-'lee-tees)

Herpes simplex
Herpes simple
('ehr-pehs 'seem-pleh)

Herpes zoster (Shingles)
Herpes zóster (Culebrilla)
('ehr-pehs 'zoh-stehr (koo-leh-'bree-yah))

Impetigo
Impétigo
(eem-'peh-tee-goh)

Pediculosis
Pediculosis
(peh-dee-koo-'loh-sees)

Glossary

Psoriasis
Psoriasis
(soh-'ree-ah-sees)

Scabies
Sarna
('sahr-nah)

Systemic lupus erythematosus
Lupus eritomatoso systémico generalizado
('loo-pohs eh-ree-toh-mah-'toh-soh sees-'teh-mee-koh)

Urticaria
Urticaria
(oor-tee-'kah-ree-ah)

➤ COMMON PROCEDURES AND DIAGNOSTICS BY SYSTEM

Head, Eye, Ear, Nose, and Throat

Audiometry
Audiometría
(ah-oo-dee-oh-meh-'tree-ah)

Color vision
Visión de color
(bee-see-'ohn deh koh-'lohr)

Refraction
Refracción
(reh-frahk-see-'ohn)

Rinne test
Examen de Rinne
(ehk-'sah-mehn deh 'ree-neh)

Romberg test
Examen de Romberg
(ehk-'sah-mehn deh 'rohm-behrg)

Smell test
Examen del olfato
(ehk-'sah-mehn dehl ohl-'fah-toh)

Snellen's test
Examen de Snellen
(ehk-'sah-mehn deh 'sneh-lehn)

Throat culture
Cultivo de garganta
(kool-'tee-boh deh gahr-'gahn-tah)

Weber's test
Examen de Weber
(ehk-'sah-mehn deh 'weh-behr)

Respiratory

Arterial blood gases
Gases arteriales
('gah-sehs ahr-teh-ree-'ah-lehs)

Bronchoscopy
Broncoscopia
(brohn-koh-'skoh-pee-ah)

Computed tomography of the chest (CT)

Tomografía axial computerizada (TAC) del pecho / tomografía axial computerizada del tórax

(toh-moh-grah-'fee-ah ahks-ee-'ahl kohm-poo-tah-ree-'sah-dah (teh ah seh) dehl 'peh-choh / toh-moh-grah-'fee-ah ahks-ee-'ahl kohm-poo-tah-ree-'sah-dah dehl 'toh-rahks)

Laryngoscopy

Laringoscopia

(lah-reen-goh-'skoh-pee-ah)

Lung biopsy

Biopsia del pulmón

(bee-'ohp-see-ah dehl pool-'mohn)

Pulmonary angiography

Angiografía pulmonar

(ahn-hee-oh-grah-'fee-ah pool-moh-'nahr)

Pulmonary function test

Examen de funcíon pulmonar

(ehk-'sah-mehn deh foon-see-'ohn pool-moh-'nahr)

Pulse oximetry

Oximetría de pulso

(ox-ee-meh-'tree-ah deh 'pool-soh)

Spiral CT of the chest

Tomografía axial computerizada (TAC) espiral del pecho

(toh-moh-grah-'fee-ah ahks-ee-'ahl kohm-poo-tah-ree-'sah-dah (teh ah seh) ehs-'pee-rahl dehl 'peh-choh)

Sputum specimen

Muestra de flema

(moo-'ehs-trah deh 'fleh-mah)

Thoracentesis
Toracentesis
(tohr-ah-sehn-'teh-sees)

Ventilation-perfusion scan (V/Q scan)
Gammagrafía de ventilación-perfusión
(gah-mee-grah-'fee-ah deh behn-tee-lah-see-'ohn pehr-foo-see-'ohn)

Cardiovascular / Peripheral Vascular

Angiogram
Angiograma
(ahn-hee-oh-'grah-mah)

Angiography
Angiografía
(ahn-hee-oh-grah-'fee-ah)

Aortogram
Aortograma
(ah-ohr-toh-'grah-mah)

Calcium
Calcio
('kahl-see-oh)

Cardiac catheterization
Cateterización cardiaca
(kah-teh-tehr-ee-sah-see-'ohn kahr-'dee-ah-kah)

Cholesterol
Colesterol
(koh-'lehs-teh-rohl)

Complete blood count
Biometría hemática
(bee-oh-meh-'tree-ah eh-'mah-tee-kah)

CPR
resucitación cardiopulmonar
(reh-soo-see-tah-see-`ohn kahr-dee-oh-pool-moh-`nahr)

Creatine kinase (CK)
Kinasa creatina
(kee-'nah-sah kreh-ah-'tee-nah)

Creatine phosphokinase (CK-MB)
Fosfokinasa creatina
(fohs-foh-kee-'nah-sah kreh-ah-'tee-nah)

Electrocardiogram
Electrocardiograma
(eh-lehk-troh-kahr-dee-oh-'grah-mah)

Erythrocyte sedimentation rate (ESR)
Índice de sedimentación de eritrocitos
('een-dee-seh deh seh-dee-mehn-tah-see-'ohn deh eh-ree-troh-'see-tohs)

Fluoroscopy
Fluoroscopía
(floo-oh-rohs-koh-'pee-ah)

Magnesium
Magnesio
(mahg-'neh-see-oh)

Potassium
Potasio
(poh-'tah-see-oh)

Serum cardiac markers
Marcadores cardiacos
(mahr-kah-'doh-rehs kahr-'dee-ah-kohs)

Serum electrolyte tests
Examen de electrolitos
(ehk-'sah-mehn deh eh-lehk-troh-'lee-tohs)

Serum lipids
Lípidos de suero
('lee-pee-dohs deh 'sweh-roh)

Sodium
Sodio
('soh-dee-oh)

Telemetry
Telemetría
(teh-leh-meh-'tree-ah)

Thallium scan
Gammagrafía de talio
(gah-mah-grah-'fee-ah deh 'tah-lee-oh)

Triglycerides
Trigliceridos
(tree-glee-seh-'ree-dohs)

Troponin
Troponina
(troh-poh-'nee-nah)

Gastrointestinal

Barium enema study
Estudio de enema de bario
(ehs-'too-dee-oh deh eh-'neh-mah deh 'bah-ree-oh)

Barium swallow
Estudio de bario
(ehs-'too-dee-oh deh 'bah-ree-oh)

Colonoscopy
Colonoscopia
(koh-lohn-ohs-'koh-pee-ah)

Computed tomography (CT) of the abdomen
Tomografia computarizada del abdomen
(toh-moh-grah-'fee-ah kohm-poo-tah-ree-'sah-dah dehl ahb-'doh-mehn)

Endoscopic retrograde cholangiopancreatography (ERCP)
Colangiopancreatografía retrógrada endoscópica (CPRE)
(koh-lahn-hee oh-pahn-kree-ah-toh-grah-'fee-ah reh-'troh-grah-dah ehn-doh-'skoh-pee-ah (seh peh 'eh-rreh eh))

Esophageal function studies
Estudio de motildad del esófago
(ehs-'too-dee-oh deh moh-teel-'dahd deh eh-'soh-fah-goh)

Esophagogastro-duodenoscopy
Esofagogastroduodenoscopia
(eh-soh-fah-goh-gahs-troh-doo-oh-dehn-oh-'skoh-pee-ah)

Examination of stool for occult blood
Examen de sangre oculta en el excremento
(ehk-'sah-mehn deh 'sahn-greh oh-'kool-tah ehn ehl ehks-kreh-'mehn-toh)

Gallbladder scan
Gammagrafía de la vesícula biliar
(gah-mah-grah-'fee-ah deh lah beh-'see-koo-lah bee-lee-'ahr)

Gastric tube analysis
Análisis de contenido gástrico
(ah-'nah-lee-sees deh kohn-teh-'nee-doh 'gahs-tree-koh)

Hepatitis studies
Estudio de hepatitis
(ehs-'too-dee-oh deh ehp-ah-'tee-tees)

Intravenous cholangiography
Colangiografía intravenosa
(koh-lahn-hee-oh-grah-'fee-ah een-trah-beh-'noh-sah)

Liver enzymes
Enzimas del hígado
(ehn-'see-mahs dehl 'ee-gah-doh)

Needle liver biopsy
Biopsia de hígado
(bee-'ohp-see-ah deh 'ee-gah-doh)

Oral cholecystography
Colecistografía oral
(koh-leh-sees-toh-grah-'fee-ah oh-'rahl)

Radioisotope liver scan
Gammagrafía nuclear del hígado
(gah-mee-grah-'fee-ah noo-kleh-'ahr dehl 'ee-gah-doh)

Serum ammonia test
Examen de amonia
(ehk-'sah-mehn deh ah-'moh-nee-ah)

Serum amylase
Amilasa
(ah-mee-'lah-sah)

Serum bilirubin test
Examen de bilirrubina
(ehk-'sah-mehn deh bee-lee-rroo-'bee-nah)

Serum lipase
Lipasa
(lee-'pah-sah)

Serum protein test
Examen de proteinas sueras
(ehk-'sah-mehn deh proh-teh-'ee-nahs 'sweh-rahs)

Sigmoidoscopy
Sigmoidoscopia
(seeg-moh-ee-doh-'skoh-pee-ah)

Stool culture
Cultivo de excremento
(kool-'tee-boh deh ehks-kreh-'mehn-toh)

Ultrasound of the biliary system
Ultrasonido del sistema biliar
(ool-trah-soh-'nee-doh dehl sees-'teh-mah bee-lee-'ahr)

Ultrasound of the gallbladder
Ultrasonido de la vesícula biliar
(ool-trah-soh-'nee-doh deh lah beh-'see-koo-lah bee-lee-'ahr)

Ultrasound of the liver
Ultrasonido del hígado
(ool-trah-soh-'nee-doh dehl 'ee-gah-doh)

Ultrasound of the pancreas
Ultrasonido del páncreas
(ool-trah-soh-'nee-doh dehl 'pahn-kree-ahs)

Upper gastrointestinal study (series)
Serie gastrointestinal
('seh-ree-eh gahs-troh-een-tehs-tee-'nahl)

Urinary/Genital

Biopsy
Biopsia
(bee-'ohp-see-ah)

Breast biopsy
Biopsia de pecho
(bee-'ohp-see-ah deh 'peh-choh)

Colposcopy
Colposcopia
(kohl-poh-'skoh-pee-ah)

Computed tomography of the kidneys
Tomografía axial computerizada (TAC) de los riñónes
(toh-moh-grah-'fee-ah ahk-see-'ahl kohm-poo-teh-ree-'sah-dah (teh ah seh) deh los ree-'nyohn-nes)

Creatinine
Creatinina
(kreh-ah-tee-'nee-nah)

Creatinine clearance
Examen de eliminación de creatinina
(ehk-'sah-mehn deh eh-lee-mee-nah-see-'ohn deh kreh-ah-tee-'nee-nah)

Dilation and curettage (D&C)
Dilatación y curetaje / raspado
(dee-lah-tah-see-'ohn ee koo-reh-'tah-heh / rahs-'pah-doh)

Intravenous pyelogram (IVP)
Pielograma intravenoso
(pee-ehl-oh-'grah-mah een-trah-beh-'noh-soh)

Kidney-ureter-bladder radiography (KUB)
Radiografía del riñón-uréter-vejiga
(rah-dee-oh-grah-'fee-ah dehl reen-'yohn oo-'reh-tehr beh-'hee-gah)

Laparascopy
Laparascopia
(lah-pah-rah-'skoh-pee-ah)

Magnetic resonance imaging (MRI)
Imagen de resonancia magnética
(ee-'mah-hehn deh reh-soh-'nahn-see-ah mahg-'neh-tee-kah)

Mammogram
Mamograma
(mah-moh-'grah-mah)

Osmolarity
Osmolaridad
(ohs-moh-lah-ree-'dahd)

Papanicolaou (pap) smear
Papanicolaou
(pah-pah-nee-koh-'lah-oh)

Pelvic ultrasound
Ultrasonido pélvico
(ool-trah-soh-'nee-doh 'pehl-bee-koh)

Pregnancy test
Prueba de embarazo
(Proo-'eh-bah deh ehm-bah-'rah-soh)

Prostate-specific antigen (PSA)
Antígeno específico de la próstata
(ahn-'tee-heh-noh ehs-peh-'see-fee-koh deh lah 'prohs-tah-tah)

Renal angiography
Angiografía renal
(ahn-hee-oh-grah-'fee-ah reh-'nahl)

Renal biopsy
Biopsia renal
(bee-'ohp-see-ah reh-'nahl)

Renal scan
Gammagrafía renal
(gah-mah-grah-'fee-ah reh-'nahl)

Renal venogram
Venograma renal
(beh-noh-'grah-mah reh-'nahl)

Retrograde pyeolography
Pielografía retrógrada
(pee-eh-loh-grah-'fee-ah reh-'troh-grah-dah)

Semen analysis
Análisis de semen
(ah-'nah-lee-sees deh 'seh-mehn)

Specific gravity
Gravidad específica
(grah-bee-'dahd ehs-peh-'see-fee-kah)

Testicular biopsy
Biopsia testicular
(bee-'ohp-see-ah tehs-tee-koo-'lahr)

Transrectal ultrasound
Ultrasonido transrectal
(ool-trah-soh-'nee-doh trahns-rehk-'tahl)

Ultrasound of the kidney
Ultrasonido del riñón
(ool-trah-soh-'nee-doh dehl reen-'yohn)

Urea nitrogen
Nitrógeno de urea
(nee-'troh-heh-noh deh oo-'reh-ah)

Urinalysis
Examen de orina
(ehk-'sah-mehn deh oh-'ree-nah)

Urodynamic studies
Estudios urodinámicos
(ehs-'too-dee-ohs oo-roh-dee-'nah-mee-kohs)

Voiding cystourethrography
Cistouretrografía
(sees-toh-oo-reh-troh-grah-'fee-ah)

Musculoskeletal

Arthrocentesis
Artrocentesis
(ahr-troh-sehn-'teh-sees)

Arthroscopy
Artroscopía
(ahr-troh-skoh-'pee-ah)

Aspiration
Aspiración
(ahs-pee-rah-see-'ohn)

Bone scan
Gammagrafía ósea / gammagrafía de hueso
(gah-mah-grah-'fee-ah 'oh-seh-ah / gah-mah-grah-'fee-ah deh 'weh-soh)

Computed axial tomography (CT)
Tomografía axial computerizada (TAC)
(toh-moh-grah-'fee-ah ahks-ee-'ahl kohm-poo-teh-ree-'sah-dah (teh ah seh))

Electromyogram
Electromiografía
(eh-lehk-troh-mee-oh-grah-'fee-ah)

Endoscopic spinal microsurgery
Microcirugía endoscópica espinal
(mee-kroh-see-roo-'hee-ah ehn-dohs-'koh-pee-kah ehs-pee-'nahl)

Magnetic resonance imaging
Resonancia magnética
(reh-soh-'nahn-see-ah mahg-'neh-tee-kah)

Myeologram
Mielograma
(mee-ehl-oh-'grah-mah)

Nuclear scanning
Gammagrafía nuclear
(gah-mah-grah-'fee-ah noo-kleh-'ahr)

Synovial fluid aspiration
Aspiración de liquido sinovial
(ahs-pee-rah-see-'ohn deh 'lee-kee-doh seen-oh-bee-'ahl)

X-rays
Rayos X
('rah-yohs 'eh-kees)

Hematologic / Lymphatic

Bone marrow aspiration
Aspiración de médula ósea
(ahs-pee-rah-see-'ohn deh 'meh-doo-lah 'oh-seh-ah)

Bone marrow biopsy
Biopsia de médula ósea
(bee-'ohp-see-ah deh 'meh-doo-lah 'oh-seh-ah)

Complete blood count
Biometria hemática
(bee-oh-'meh-tree-ah eh-'mah-tee-kah)

Erythrocyte indices
Indices de eritrocitos
('een-dee-sehs deh eh-ree-troh-'see-tohs)

Lymphangiography
Linfangiografía
(leen-fahn-hee-oh-grah-'fee-ah)

Peripheral smear
Frote sanguíneo
('froh-teh sahn-'hee-neh-oh)

Endocrine

Blood glucose
Nivel de azúcar en la sangre
(nee-'behl deh ah-'soo-kahr ehn lah 'sahn-greh)

Computed tomography (CT)
Tomografía axial computerizada
(toh-moh-grah-'fee-ah ahk-see-'ahl kohm-poo-tehr-ee-'sah-dah)

Cranial radiography
Radiografía de cráneo
(rah-dee-oh-grah-'fee-ah deh 'krah-nee-oh)

Fasting blood glucose
Nivel de azúcar en la sangre en ayunas
(nee-'behl deh ah-'soo-kahr ehn lah 'sahn-greh ehn ah-'yoo-nahs)

Free thyroxine (Free T4)
Tiroxina libre
(tee-rohks-'ee-nah 'lee-breh)

Glycosylated hemoglobin (Hb A1c)
Hemoglobina glicosilada
(eh-moh-gloh-'bee-nah glee-koh-see-'lah-dah)

Growth hormone level
Nivel de hormona de crecimiento
(nee-'behl deh ohr-'moh-nah deh kreh-see-mee-'ehn-toh)

Magnetic resonance imaging
Imagen de resonancia magnética
(ee-'mah-hehn deh rreh-soh-'nahn-see-ah mahg-'neh-tee-kah)

Glossary

Oral glucose tolerance test

Examen de tolerancia a la glucosa oral

(ehk-'sah-mehn deh toh-leh-'rahn-see-ah ah lah gloo-'koh-sah oh-'rahl)

Random blood glucose

Nivel de azúcar en la sangre al azar

(nee-'behl deh ah-'soo-kahr ehn lah 'sahn-greh ahl ah-'sahr)

Serum insulin

Nivel de insulina

(nee-'behl deh een-soo-'lee-nah)

Serum thyroxine (T4)

Tiroxina (T4)

(tee-rohks-'ee-nah (teh 'kwah-troh))

Serum triiodothyronine (T3)

Triiodotironina (T3)

(tree-ee-oh-doh-tee-roh-'nee-nah (teh trehs))

Thyroid scan

Gammagrafía de la tiroides

(gah-mah-grah-'fee-ah deh lah tee-'roh-ee-dehs)

Thyroid-stimulating hormone (TSH)

Hormona estimulante de la tiroide

(ohr-'moh-nah ehs-tee-moo-'lahn-teh deh lah tee-'roh-ee-dehs)

Urine ketones

Ketonas en la orina

(keh-'toh-nahs ehn lah oh-'ree-nah)

Neurologic

Angiogram
Angiograma
(ehn-'hee-oh-grah-mah)

Brain scan
Gammagrafía del cerebro / imagen del cerebro
(gah-mah-grah-'fee-ah dehl seh-'reh-broh / ee-'mah-hehn dehl seh-'ree-broh)

Carotid duplex
Examen de la carótida (con ultrasonido y Doppler)
(ehk-'sah-mehn deh lah kah-'roh-tee-dah kohn ool-trah-soh-'nee-doh ee 'doh-plehr)

Computed tomography (CT) of the skull
Tomografía axial computerizada (TAC) del cráneo
(toh-moh-grah-'fee-ah kohm-poo-teh-ree-'sah-dah dehl 'krah-neh-oh (teh ah seh))

Echoencephalogram
Ecoencefalograma
(eh-koh-ehn-seh-fah-loh-'grah-mah)

Electroencephalogram
Electroencefalograma
(eh-lehk-troh-ehn-seh-fah-loh-'grah-mah)

Electromyogram
Electromiograma
(eh-lehk-troh-mee-oh-'grah-mah)

Glasgow coma scale
Escala de coma de Glasgow
(ehs-'kah-lah deh 'koh-mah deh 'glahs-gow)

Glossary

Lumbar puncture
Punción lumbar
(poon-see-'ohn loom-'bahr)

Magnetic resonance angiography (MRA)
Angiografía de resonancia magnética (MRA)
(ahn-hee-oh-grah-'fee-ah deh reh-soh-'nahn-see-ah mahg-'neh-tee-kah ('ehm-eh 'eh-reh ah))

Magnetic resonance imaging (MRI)
Imagen de resonancia magnética (IRM)
(ee-'mah-hehn deh res-soh-'nahn-see-ah mahg-'neh-tee-kah (ee 'eh-reh 'ehm-eh))

Myelogram
Mielograma
(mee-ehl-oh-'grah-mah)

Positron emission tomography (PET)
Tomografía de emisión de positrones (PET)
(toh-moh-grah-'fee-ah deh eh-mee-see-'ohn deh poh-see-'troh-nehs (peh eh teh))

Dermatologic

Antinuclear antibody (ANA)
Anticuerpo antinuclear
(ahn-tee-'kwehr-poh ahn-tee-noo-kleh-'ahr)

Coagulation studies
Estudios de coagulación
(ehs-'too-dee-ohs deh koh-ah-goo-lah-see-'ohn)

Complete blood count
Biometria hemática
(bee-oh-meh-'tree-ah eh-'mah-tee-kah)

Coomb's test
Examen de Coomb
(ehk-'sah-mehn deh coomb)

C-reactive protein (CRP)
Proteina reactiva C
(pro-teh-'ee-nah reh-ahk-'tee-bah seh)

DNA antibody
Anticuerpo DNA
(ahn-tee-'kwehr-poh eh 'eh-neh ah)

Drainage culture
Cultivo de drenaje
(kool-'tee-boh deh dreh-'nah-heh)

Erythrocyte sedimentation rate (ESR)
Índice de sedimentación de eritrocitos
('een-dee-seh deh seh-dee-mehn-tah-see-'ohn deh eh-ree-troh-'see-tohs)

Gram stain
Tinción de Gram
(teen-see-'ohn deh grahm)

Rapid plasma reagin (RPR)
Reagina plasmática rápida
(reh-ah-'heh-nah plahs-'mah-tee-kah 'rah-pee-dah)

Renal biopsy
Biopsia renal
(bee-'ohp-see-ah reh-'nahl)

Rheumatoid factor (RF)
Factor reumatico
('fahk-tohr reh-oo-'mah-tee-koh)

Sedimentation rate
Índice de sedimentación
('een-dee-seh deh seh-dee-mehn-tah-see-'ohn)

Serum immunoglobulin E (IgE)
Inmunoglobulina E
(een-moo-noh-gloh-boo-'lee-nah eh)

Skin biopsy
Biopsia de piel
(bee-'ohp-see-ah deh pee-'ehl)

Urinalysis
Examen de orina
(ehk-'sah-mehn deh oh-'ree-nah)

Wood's lamp
Lámpara de Wood
('lahm-pah-rah deh wood)

Wound culture
Cultivo de herida
(kool-'tee-boh deh eh-'ree-dah)

Specialists

Anesthetist
anestesista
(ah-nehs-teh-`sees-tah)

Assistant
ayudante
(ah-yoo-`dahn-teh)

Bacteriologist
bacteriólogo
(bahk-teh-ree-`oh-loh-goh)

Case Manager
gestoro de caso
(hes-tor-o deh cah-so)

Dietician
dietista
(dee-eh-`tees-tah)

Gynecologist
ginecólogo
(hee-neh-`koh-loh-goh)

Obstetrician
obstetriz
(ohb-steh-`trees)

Pharmacist
farmacéutico
(fahr-mah-`seh-oo-tee-koh)

Technician
técnico
(`tehk-nee-koh)

Therapist
terapeuta
(the-rah-peh-`oo-tah)

Orderly
practicante
(prahk-tee-`kahn-teh)

Glossary

Radiologist
radiólogo
(rah-dee-`oh-loh-goh)

Social worker
trabajador social
(trah-bah-hah-`dohr soh-see-`ahl)

➤ *COMMON SURGERIES BY SYSTEM*

Head, Eye, Ear, Nose, and Throat

Adenoidectomy
Adeinoidectomía
(ah-dee-ehn-oh-ee-dehk-toh-'mee-ah)

Cochlear implant
Implante de coclea
(eem-'plahn-teh deh koh-'kleh-ah)

Enucleation
Enucleación
(eh-noo-kleh-ah-see-'ohn)

Keratoplasty
Queratoplastia
(keh-rah-toh-'plahs-tee-ah)

Myringotomy
Miringotomía
(mee-reen-goh-toh-'mee-ah)

Nasal packing
Empaque nasal
(ehm-'pah-keh nah-'sahl)

Nasal polypectomy
Polipectomía nasal
(poh-lee-pehk-toh-'mee-ah nah-'sahl)

Nasoseptoplasty
Nasoseptoplastia
(nah-soh-sehp-toh-'plahs-tee-ah)

Partial laryngectomy
Laringectomía parcial
(lah-reen-hehk-toh-'mee-ah pahr-see-'ahl)

Photocoagulation
Fotocoagulación
(foh-toh-koh-ah-gool-ah-see-'ohn)

Radical neck dissection
Disección radical de cuello
(dee-sehk-see-'ohn rah-dee-'kahl de 'kweh-yoh)

Septum repair
Reparación del septo
(reh-pah-rah-see-'ohn dehl 'sehp-toh)

Stapedectomy
Estribectomía
(eh-stree-behk-toh-'mee-ah)

Tonsillectomy
Tonsilectomía
(tohn-see-lehk-toh-'mee-ah)

Total laryngectomy
Laringectomía total
(lah-reen-hehk-toh-'mee-ah toh-'tahl)

Tympanoplasty
Timpanoplastia
(teem-pah-noh-'plahs-tee-ah)

Vitrectomy
Vitreotomia
(bee-treh-oh-toh-'mee-ah)

Respiratory

Chest tube insertion
Inserción de tubo torácico / toracostomía
(een-sehr-see-'ohn deh 'too-boh toh-'rah-see-koh / toh-rah-koh-stoh-'mee-ah)

Lung biopsy
Biopsia de pulmón
(bee-'ohp-see-ah deh pool-'mohn)

Lung resection
Resección de pulmón
(reh-sehk-see-'ohn deh pool-'mohn)

Mediastinoscopy
Mediastinoscopia
(meh-dee-ahs-tee-noh-'skoh-pee-ah)

Cardiovascular / Peripheral

Cardiac transplant
Transplante cardiaco
(trahns-'plahn-teh kahr-'dee-ah-koh)

Coronary artery bypass graft (CABG)
Injerto y derivación de arteria coronaria
(een-'hehr-toh ee deh-ree-bah-see-'ohn deh ahr-'teh-ree-ah koh-roh-'nah-ree-ah)

Endarterectomy
Endarterectomía
(ehn-dahr-tehr-ehk-toh-'mee-ah)

Pacemaker placement
Instalación de marcapasos
(een-stah-lah-see-'ohn deh mahr-kah-'pah-sohs)

Stent placement
Inserción de stent
(een-sehr-see-'ohn deh stehnt)

Varicotomy
Varicotomía
(bahr-ee-koh-toh-'mee-ah)

Vein ligation
Ligadura de vena
(lee-gah-'doo-rah deh 'beh-nah)

Gastrointestinal

Appendectomy
Apendectomía / extirpación del apéndice
(ah-pehn-dehk-toh-'mee-ah / ehks-teer-pah-see-'ohn dehl ah-'pehn-dee-seh)

Cholecystectomy
Colecistectomía
(koh-leh-sees-tehk-toh-'mee-ah)

Colostomy
Colostomía
(koh-lohs-toh-'mee-ah)

Esophagogastrectomy
Esofagogastrectomía
(eh-soh-fah-goh-gahs-trehk-toh-'mee-ah)

Gastrojejunostomy
Gastrojejunostomía
(gahs-troh-heh-hoo-nohs-toh-'mee-ah)

Gastrostomy
Gastrostomía
(gahs-troh-stoh-'mee-ah)

Hernia repair
Reparación de hernia
(reh-pah-rah-see-'ohn deh 'ehr-nee-ah)

Ileoanal anastomosis
Anastomosis ileoanal
(ah-nahs-toh-'moh-sees ee-lee-oh-ah-'nahl)

Ileostomy
Ileostomía
(ee-lee-oh-stoh-'mee-ah)

Proctocolectomy
Proctocolectomía
(prohk-toh-koh-lehk-toh-'mee-ah)

Pyloroplasty
Piloroplastia
(pee-lohr-oh-'plahs-tee-ah)

Tumor resection
Resección de tumor
(reh-sehk-see-'ohn deh too-'mohr)

Vagotomy
Vagotomía
(bah-goh-toh-'mee-ah)

Urinary / Genital

Kidney transplant
Transplante de riñón
(trahns-'plahn-teh deh reen-'yohn)

Nephrostomy
Nefrostomía
(neh-frohs-toh-'mee-ah)

Musculoskeletal

Laparoscopic surgery
Cirugía laparoscópica
(see-roo-'hee-ah lah-pah-rohs-'koh-pee-kah)

Total hip replacement
Reemplazo de cadera total
(reh-ehm-'plah-soh deh kah-'deh-rah toh-'tahl)

Total knee replacement
Reemplazo de rodilla total
(reh-ehm-'plah-soh deh roh-'dee-yah toh-'tahl)